BIG AND STRONG
WITHOUT STEROIDS

YURIY OLIYNYK DPT, CSCS, PES

ISBN-13: 978-1-9830-1084-2

I would like to thank **Diana Oliynyk** for helping her artistically challenged father to put this book together

bigandstrongapp@gmail.com
www.bigandstrongapp.com

Table of Contents

INTRODUCTION

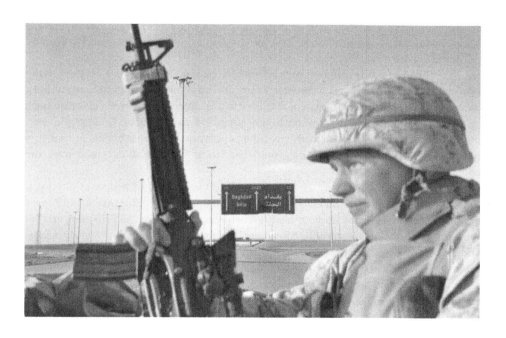

"How you do anything is how you do everything."
— T. Harv Eker

One look at the Mr. Olympia lineup should make it very clear that every single one of today's pros takes massive amounts of anabolic steroids. It would be naïve to think that things are much different in powerlifting or weightlifting. Now, add to that the lifestyle where all these guys do is train, eat and sleep. That's their job! Compare it to the lives of the rest of us with work, school, kids and everything else. It should be obvious that copying training programs of these champions by your regular guy is as absurd as trying to live the life of Bill Gates while earning a minimum wage.

Taking steroids is a personal choice and it should be an easy one to make. Let's be honest guys: unless you are a professional bodybuilder, nobody really cares about your muscles. Only teenage girls will fall for a guy with the biggest biceps. But once you are out of high school you better have more than that. So why take steroids? So you could have big muscles few years earlier? And then what? What is the sense of accomplishment? You took load of drugs and now you are so huge you can barely scratch your ass. Congratulations! It's like buying a medal at a souvenir store and thinking you are a real champion.

Obviously, it is different for professional bodybuilders. They earn their living by the way they look and, with the way things are, have no choice but to take steroids. I am sure they don't particularly enjoy this situation. Even here, however, the damage is undeniable. Bodybuilding contests are supposed to be about finding the best physiques on Earth. Yet 99% of the world's population will probably agree that it is no longer the case. None of this would happen if steroids didn't take over the bodybuilding.

Aside from the pros, there are generally two groups of people at any gym. The first group are what you could call recreational members. They are mostly there because exercising is good for your health. They are normally casually roaming around the gym while socializing heavily. They usually know that flexing elbow works biceps and bench press is for pecs. Anything much more complicated than that has no interest to them. They are probably not the ones reading this book.

The second group is a more serious part of the gym population. Some of them are your typical hardcore lifters. These are normally the guys that always have a hood on and carry a gallon of water for some reason. They usually describe their training style as "old school." It is difficult to know for sure what they mean by that.

But then there are people who need the results. Not necessarily because they want to compete in bodybuilding or powerlifting. They just need to know what to do and why they are doing it. These are the guys that usually have some rationale behind their training program. They don't always know what they are doing but at least they are trying to make sense of things.

The problem is that while this group is figuring it all out, lots of time can be wasted. And we are not talking about weeks or months here. The number of possible combinations of all training variables is virtually unlimited. Expecting to figure out what is best for you based on intuition alone is as realistic as flying into space in random direction while hopping to arrive at some specific star constellation. Dorian Yates has a famous quote on this subject: "if I listened to my instincts, I'd be down at the pub chasing women, not under 400-pound bar squatting."

When I just started training in early 90-s back in Ukraine there was a very limited amount of literature about resistance training. Bodybuilding and powerlifting were not Olympic sports and, therefore, were not recognized in USSR. The only relevant sources we had was the Weightlifting literature. It was difficult to understand for a teenager because Soviet training books were always very academic. But in the way, that situation was a blessing: it taught us all to appreciate knowledge. When books and magazines finally started getting through, we all would jump on them like they were made of gold. We would read them from cover to cover and then discuss the material for weeks.

Now the situation is the opposite. The amount of information about training is almost infinite. More than anyone can get through in a lifetime. Anyone can just open their phone and learn anything and everything about training. But they don't. We are so spoiled with all this knowledge that it made us ignorant. We would rather show up at the gym and wing it.

Those who do try to research the topic end up drowning in all the information available. How do you know where to start? How do you know that the source is reliable? Some guy on YouTube looks legit. But he looks like he is on steroids himself. Does that mean that his recommendations only work on steroids? Is there the fine print that I am missing?

This is not to say that there are no good books about training. They do exist. The problem is that some of them are so overly scholarly that even someone experienced will have trouble getting through. Classics such as "Science and Practice of Strength Training" and "Supertraining" come to mind immediately and, if you ever came across them, you know exactly what I am talking about. How can you expect a high school kid who wants to get in shape for the summer to be able to extract anything out of them?

Some might think that hiring a professional might be the answer. But do consider the fact that there are currently no official licensing requirements for personal trainers. Anyone can declare to be one at any moment. Next thing you know someone who was an accountant a week ago has you swinging kettlebells on the Bosu ball.

That's not to say that all personal trainers are useless. But your chances of hiring a trainer that is actually competent are about as high as if you were playing the lottery. The only difference is that playing the lottery would be a lot cheaper. It is truly outrageous how much some of these "experts" charge for their services.

And even if you did get lucky with a knowledgeable trainer that you could afford, do you really need someone to babysit you at the gym? For example, do you call a nutritionist to come over every time you have a meal? Of course not. You can hire one for a consultation but for the most part you should know how to properly feed yourself. Wouldn't it be nice if the same thinking was applied to training? Even though not many of us are NASCAR level drivers, most people know how to drive. Similarly, you don't need to be qualified to coach our national weightlifting team, but you should still have a basic idea of how to keep yourself fit.

It is interesting that understanding the essentials of exercising and nutrition is not considered to be important part of general education. Somehow knowing that $a^2+b^2=c^2$ is given a higher priority. US government spends all this money on promoting a healthy lifestyle, but what does really mean? Do guidelines about how many minutes of physical activity someone should perform per week really help anybody? Because that's what you will find if you look up current exercise recommendations from the Department of Health. We are planning missions to Mars and yet there is no credible explicit exercise manual available to public. I hope this book is a step in that direction.

I am not suggesting blindly following this training system. This book is not intended as all-inclusive encyclopedia. Read and learn about resistance training as much as possible. Books by Mark Rippetoe and Stuart McRobert are good choices once you are done with this one. There are many other good sources of information available and it will take you some years to put it all together. In the meantime use a solid training plan such as "Big and Strong." I guarantee you, the more you learn about training, the more this system will make sense to you.

Some of you might be a little alarmed by the negative tone of this intro, but I don't like to dance around the issue. The sport that has been the biggest passion of my life is back in Stone Age. Steroids started all the confusion and social media keeps adding to it. I can't make officials to implement mandatory drug testing, just like I can't remove all absurd information from the Internet. All I can do is to show how you can achieve more than you thought was possible at the gym without ever messing with needles. Maybe it's not too late to swing the tide in the positive direction.

BIOLOGY

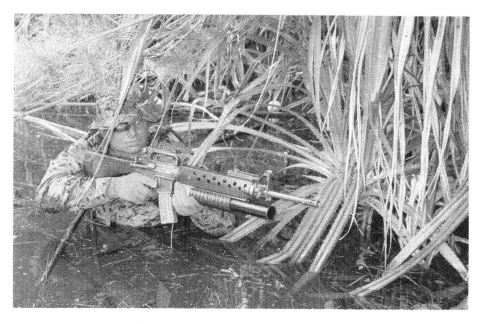

"What doesn't kill you makes you stronger."
    - Friedrich Nietzsche

This section will be a brief overview of human anatomy and physiology. We will mostly focus on systems that work in conjunction with muscles. People with medical background might find this discussion a bit rudimentary and can skip over to the next section. For the rest of the readers this information should provide some basic understanding of human body functioning and how it is related to training. Just keep in mind that drawings included in this chapter are schematic representations and don't necessarily resemble the appearance of the actual organs. If you want to dive deeper into this topic "Essentials of Strength Training and Conditioning" is your best friend.

Musculoskeletal system

Muscles are composed of multiple muscle cells (fibers) grouped together in one unit. Muscles are attached to the *bones* by *tendons*. Injury to a tendon is referred to as a *strain*. When muscle contracts it shortens its length and pulls the bones it is attached to together. The place where two bones meet is called a *joint*. Adjacent bones are often connected together by *ligament* to prevent excessive movement. Injury to a ligament is referred to as a *sprain*. The surface of the bone at the joint is covered with smooth connective tissue called *cartilage*. Its purpose is to decrease the friction between bones during movement. Wearing out of cartilage leads to pathologic condition called *osteoarthritis*.

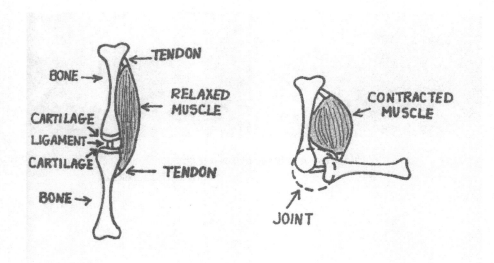

Main muscle groups

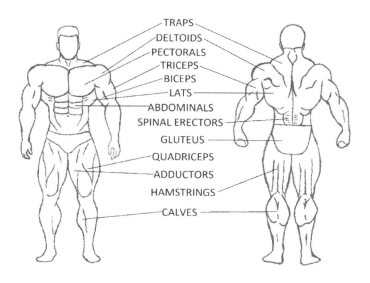

TRAPS
DELTOIDS
PECTORALS
TRICEPS
BICEPS
LATS
ABDOMINALS
SPINAL ERECTORS
GLUTEUS
QUADRICEPS
ADDUCTORS
HAMSTRINGS
CALVES

Neuromuscular system

Voluntary muscle activation is initiated at the motor cortex of the *brain*. It then travels down through the *spinal cord* and reaches muscles by respective motor *neurons*. Groups of neurons traveling together are called *nerves*. Each muscle is innervated by multiple motor neurons. One motor neuron can innervate multiple muscle fibers (referred to as a *motor unit*). The number of motor units activated simultaneously is one of the factor determining the strength of the muscle contraction.

The bigger the muscle the stronger the contraction it is theoretically capable of. This is why the easiest way to get stronger is to become bigger. However, people with the biggest muscles (bodybuilders, for example) are not always the strongest. The reason for such discrepancy lies in the ability to recruit maximum number of motor units at the same time. This is why in order to develop a muscle to its maximum potential both increasing the size (hypertrophy) of individual muscle fibers and the ability to simultaneously activate as many of them as possible have to be addressed.

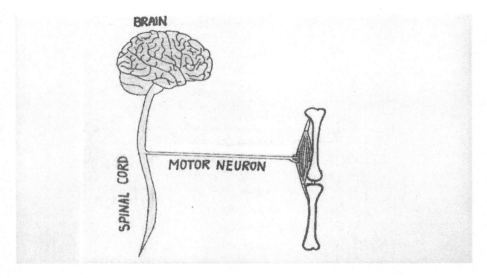

Metabolism

Just like any machinery, our muscles require fuel to perform work. Food we consume serves as a source of such fuel. Once it is digested in the *gastrointestinal tract* and absorbed into the bloodstream, it is available for utilization. There are two main ways our body converts food into energy: anaerobic (without O_2) and aerobic (with O_2). *Anaerobic* pathway is capable of quickly producing large amount of energy (for example, weightlifters lifting maximum load) but cannot be sustained for long time. On the other hand, *aerobic* pathway is unable to provide instant source of high energy, however, can be utilized for prolonged periods of time (walking, for example). Most activities will fall in between of the two examples mentioned here and will involve both pathways simultaneously. The degree to which each pathway will contribute to the overall energy production will depend on the intensity of the activity.

Cardiovascular system

As was stated earlier, muscles need nutrients and oxygen to operate. *Blood* serves as a transporter of these substances to muscles and also to carry CO_2 and other waste products away from the muscle. Blood is being pumped through the body by the *heart*. Once the blood enters the heart it is sent to the *lungs* where CO_2 is exchanged for O_2. Vessels that carry blood full of CO_2 to the heart are called *veins*. Vessels that carry oxygenated blood from the heart to the rest of the body are called *arteries*.

Ability to sustain continuous work of relatively high intensity is referred to as **endurance**. It is closely related to efficiency of cardiovascular system to provide O_2 to working muscles and removing CO_2 and other by-products of metabolism away from them. The main adaptation that takes place as a result of endurance type of training is the increased ability of the heart to pump blood (*cardiac output*).

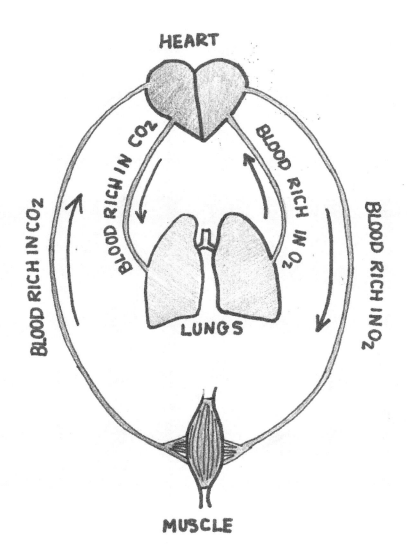

THEORY

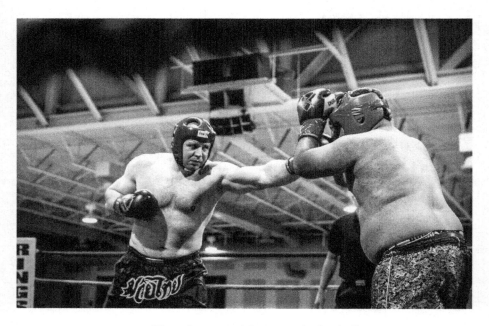

"You miss 100% of shoots you don't take."
– Wayne Gretzky

The purpose of this book is to give clear training guidelines that will produce results without using performance enhancing drugs (PEDs). It is still necessary to have some basic understanding of the principles behind the actual recommendations. Think of these as "10 commandments" that will guide your gym life, regardless of the training approach you ultimately decide to choose.

The material covered in this chapter is quite complicated. I will try to do my very best to present it in the simplest way possible. Those interested in more in-depth explanation I invite to check out "Big and Strong" YouTube channel.

It is good to be open-minded but it is also important to have critical mindset. Fitness industry is currently flooded with misleading information and we are not so lucky to let the research give us all the answers. Unfortunately modern sports science academia is preoccupied with randomizes controlled trials that mostly produce evidence for what are mostly well known facts.

For example, have you ever heard someone questioning the effectiveness of muay thai due to lack of peer reviewed meta-analysis? Or does a black belt at legitimate jiu-jitsu school have to produce some 8 week study with 25 college students to be considered an expert? My point is that some things are just simply too complex to be studied by "A causes B" experiment.

Which does not mean that we all are just stumbling in the darkness and it's time to turn to witchcraft. This chapter will give you concrete tools to separate garbage from effective training guidelines. I encourage you to start applying this knowledge by analyzing training programs presented later in this book.

Adaptation

Adaptation is the cornerstone of any training methodology. It is the ability of human organism to change in order to adjust to the demands placed on it. The classic analogy that is being used to explain adaptation is tanning. This darkening of the skin is a protective mechanism with which our bodies adapt to a regular sun exposure.

In order to produce an adaptation the stimulus must fall within a specific range. If you stay in the sun for a minute, for example, not much will probably happen. Just like doing one push-up will not turn you into a Hulk. On the other hand, if you jump right to sunbathing for an hour, a sunburn might occur. This would be an equivalent of getting injured while attempting a load is way too heavy.

Another thing we have to take into account is that adaptation process is not random. There is a cause (sun rays) and effect (skin pigmentation). In regards to training it means that in order to produce a desired effect, APPROPRIATE training stimulus must be selected. This is why you don't start yoga in order to grow your biceps or don't do barbell curls if you want to lose weight.

Supercompensation

The following discussion is an interpretation of Selye's general adaptation syndrome theory, modified to how it relates to training. Let's imagine Yuriy, who has never done any resistance training (point A), decided to get stronger. He goes to the gym and lifts 20 pounds 10 times.

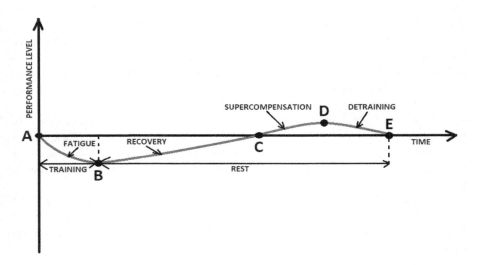

After the first training session (point B) Yuriy's performance abilities will decrease. This is due to the fatigue accumulated during the workout. If sufficient amount of rest is allowed and all the necessary nutrients are provided, Yuriy will eventually be able to go back to the previous level of performance (point C). But now that he has been subjected to a new form of stress (training), his body will try to prepare itself just in case this happens again (point D).

The difference between points A and D is called supercompensation. It is the desired effect we try to elicit by subjecting ourselves to various training protocols. Similarly to how once a broken bone heals it becomes stronger, our muscles become more resilient after training stimulus was administered.

Another important point illustrated here is that for the supercompensation to occur, the recovery has to take place first. Ideally you want to have every training session at point D. This applies to an athlete as a whole and different individual structures in particular. For example, after training biceps on Monday you might still feel fresh enough for a back workout on Tuesday. However, since the biceps get utilized during a lot of back exercises, such poor planning could impede the progress for both of these muscle groups.

Achieving complete recovery before each training session is not always possible. This is because different muscles and different physiological systems require various amount of time for full recuperation. Still care must be taken to plan everything as OPTIMALLY as possible. Chronic violations of proper recovery process could eventually lead to the state of **overtraining**. Such condition should not be confused with simply being very tired. The more accurate way to look at overtraining is as situation similar to our sunburn analogy: in both instances significant time away from the stressor will be necessary to allow the body to heal.

On the other hand, if too much time elapses between training sessions, detraining might take place. Your body will not retain a new acquired ability if it is no longer useful. As they say: if you don't use it, you lose it. Similarly to how your tan fades away if you avoid the sun long enough, the "gains" will disappear (point E) if too much rest is given.

Progressive overload

Since now the performance level of humble Yuriy has increased (point D), lifting 20 pounds 10 times will not be as challenging at the next training session. Therefore, the magnitude of supercompensation will be smaller, if any. You couldn't just tan for 10 minutes at a time for infinite number of days and expect your skin to get darker every time. Similarly, in order to elicit continuous adaptation training stimulus has to increase over time.

There are two main ways for Yuriy to increase how demanding the session is: increase the volume (total number of sets and reps performed) and increase the intensity (the weight lifted). Increasing volume has its place to a certain extent. After certain point, however, number of reps will be in hundreds and the training will resemble a marathon. One look at distance runners should make it clear that this is not the best way to get big and strong.

On the other hand, if you look at sports such as shot put or strongman, the relationship between strength and size is rather obvious. As a result, moving towards higher training poundages is considered to be a preferred direction of progressive overload for our purposes.

Progressive overload rate has to be balances with recovery capabilities. It takes time for muscle proteins to be synthesized and for neural pathways to become more efficient. If you increase weight before adequate adaptation occurs, your lifting technique will start to deteriorate. Now, instead of getting bigger and stronger, you are wearing out you joints and slowly progressing towards injury.

Specificity

The easiest way to think of specificity is as efficiency. Let's use example of sweeping the room. There are multiple ways to go about. One could decide to use broom to do it, while someone else might decide to choose a toothbrush. It's not that it is impossible to complete this task with the toothbrush, but most people would find it to be obvious that the using the broom is way more effective.

Similar thing happens at the gym. People always ask if they have to squat, for example. Well, you don't really have to. Do the leg extensions if that's what your heart desires. Just be mindful that it might take you 20-30 years to develop decent quads with leg extensions, while it could be accomplished in 2 or 3 with squats.

People often have over exaggerated sense of sacrifice when it comes to finding time to exercise in their "busy" schedule. Yet when they actually make it to the gym, they feel completely fine wasting their "precious" time doing the most unproductive things imaginable. Would you invest your savings into a bank that doesn't offer reasonable interest rate? Then why invest your time and effort into ineffective training methodology?

Specificity is always goal specific. What is a good tool for sweeping the floor, might not be as efficient for brushing your teeth. Likewise, what is good training regimen for someone preparing to run a marathon, most likely will not be as effective for someone getting ready for arm wrestling competition. This is why *it is very important to have a clear idea of what is to be accomplished at the gym.* Properly set goals give your training direction. Otherwise training becomes equivalent to trading water: you are expending energy but not really going anywhere.

Energy budget

Following the above discussion, one might ask why not to perform both squat and leg extensions? Let me explain. Imagine that your payday is in a week and you barely have enough money to feed yourself. What would be the mature thing to do? Most likely you would try to get the most bang for your buck and stack up with food staples such as bread, eggs, milk, etc. Anything more fancy than that and you will end up struggling towards the end of the week.

Similar thinking has to be applied at the gym. Our "energy budget" is limited and it doesn't change that much over time. Therefore, the more energy you spend on some exotic exercise you saw on Instagram, the less you will have on your bread and butter training.

Anyone can blast away at the gym for a week or even a month. Supersets and forced reps. Screaming and moaning. Your pre-workout energy drink is kicking in. A pretty girl exercising nearby is watching. You feel like Rocky Balboa! The problem is that in the process so much recovery debt will be created that for the following few months you will be running on empty tank. Most of such overly enthusiastic (or rather inpatient) gym members will usually disappear during this time. It is the same as if you took the money you had to feed yourself for a week and blew it all at the club to impress your friends. It might feel good at the moment, but the rest of the week won't be as awesome.

How large your "energy budget" is depends on how much food and sleep you get. We'll cover nutrition later on. As far as the sleep, the norm for most people is in 7-9 hours range. Intense training will probably put you on the higher end. Also, take into account the use of PEDs when comparing your training regimen to the one of your favorite IFBB pro.

Another factor that has to be considered when you balance your training with recovery is your life outside of the gym. If you have physically demanding job, the training programs presented here might need to be modified (fancy term for this is *autoregulation*). For example, if you feel that you are not recovering between training sessions, reduce the number of sets in some exercises or even remove them altogether. Just like constant spending more money than you earn will result in bankruptcy, *continuously training more than you can recover from will result in overtraining.*

The bottom line is that we always managing limited time and energy. This applies for both professional athletes and amateurs. The difference between these groups is that pros have much larger "budget" at their disposal and, therefore, can "afford" a lot more training. Regardless of the circumstances, achieving the best results with the resources available is the primary purpose of an effective programming.

Accommodation

Let's go back to the analogy of sweeping the room. Imagine that you swept your room and were able to remove 75% of all the dirt. If you decided to do it again, you would probably get rid of additional 15%. And the next time you would only receive 5% for your effort. Therefore, even though you keep putting the same amount of work (sweeping the room), the outcome you are getting for it decreases over time. As a result, the difference in cleanness of the room after it was swept 50 times and 100 times would be negligible. This phenomena is called the law of diminishing returns and the same thing happens in the gym. Doing the same thing over and over will eventually stop working.

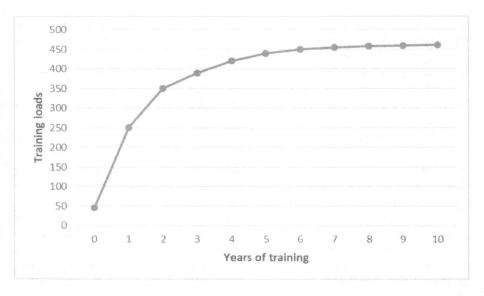

Another lesson to be learned here that the rate of your progress at the gym will inevitably decrease. It is generally pretty easy to increase bench press from 50 pounds to a 100, but going from 500 to 550 is a different story. If you wanted to continue to increase the cleanness of the room from the above example, your approach eventually would have to resemble a sterilization process. Similarly, the more advanced you become the more precise your training prescription must be. The more diligent you have to become in regards to your diet and sleep. Shortcuts you got away with as a beginner, might become disastrous at the elite level.

Variation

Due to the accommodation some variation is required to make sure our muscles don't get "bored" with training. It is important, however, not to get so out there in the process that now you are sweeping the room with a toothbrush (remember about specificity). For example, TheraBand pull-aparts would probably not be the best substitution for pull-ups. On the other hand, changing the grip width or the number of reps per set would be a lot better choice.

Some might say that all we need is to change the order of exercises "to keep muscles guessing." In reality, however, things are a little more complicated. Even if we rotate different exercises during training (*muscle confusion* training principle), the overall physiological stimuli remains relatively unchanged from session to session. It is unlikely that our endocrine system will be able to detect the difference if you simply switched from dumbbell curls to barbell curls. This might not be very important if you supplement with steroids. But for those of us who rely on natural production of testosterone such details are everything.

Preplanned variability of training is your basic definition of ***periodization***. Its various forms will be presented later on. Other ways to change up your training will also be discussed in the "Intermediate level" section. Only at this time variation starts to become important. Beginners will be able to grow by simply following a basic template (it takes some time for the process of accommodation to set in).

It is imperative not to get carried away with all the substitutions and modifications. Switching too many exercises and other parameters will make training process too chaotic. It will be difficult to tell if you are actually improving from session to session or you are simply doing something different every time. The point of employing variation is to ensure progress, not entertainment.

Transformation

Transformation is all about how improvement in one exercise affects your performance in other exercises. Its implication is what allows the use of variability. Obviously, the more similar exercises are the higher degree of transfer there will be. For example, if your front squat increased be 50 pounds you can expect a significant improvement in the back squat as well. On the other hand, equal improvement in leg press will not affect your back squat to a similar degree.

This process is not immediate (that's why term "delayed transformation" is often used). It takes time and proper planning to transform one athletic quality into another. For example, increasing your shoulder press by 100 pounds is expected to have at least some positive effect on your bench press. But it doesn't mean that the next time you are doing bench press you can just bump the weight up by 100 pounds. It simply implies that your improvement in shoulder press create a foundation for a POTENTIAL progress in the bench press. This is another reason why changing exercises from session to session (method called *muscle confusion*) is not the most effective approach. It simply never allows for full transformation to take place.

Muscle memory

"Muscle memory" is normally being used in reference to our ability to retain motor skills. For example, once you learn how to swim you will always remember it. In resistance training this term is also used to describe the ability of our muscles to return to their peak size and strength rather easily. Let's imagine that after a year of training you were able to deadlift 500 pounds. But then your wife had triplets and the gym was out of question for the following few months. Obviously during that time all your gym progress will be lost (due to "detraining"). Surprisingly enough, when you get back to lifting it will not take you another twelve months to get back to deadlifting 500 pounds. It will probably happen in one or two months. Muscle memory is to be thanked for it.

The point of this discussion is not to give you an excuse for excessive gym absenteeism. Understanding of muscle memory concept combined with transformation should help you further comprehend bases of periodization. Let's look at the following example. Imagine you decided to focus on powerlifting for a few months and temporarily removed all the isolation exercises from your program. Due to lack of direct training, after few weeks your arms might appear to lose some size. This is quite concerning considering that it took a lot of effort to add those couple of inches. But then you remember that because of muscle memory getting them back won't be nearly as difficult as to grow them initially. Deep breath.

Now let's add transformation to this discussion. Imagine that during those few months of powerlifting-only training you added 40 pounds to your bench and military presses. Both of those exercises involve elbow extension, therefore, at least some of that progress is expected to carry over into your triceps training. As a result, not only these few months will not cause a permanent decrease of the size of your "guns," but they will actually set stage for new growth spurt once direct arm training is resumed.

Individualization

Perhaps the most misunderstood aspect of training process. I firmly believe that increased importance of individualization in recent couple of decades is caused by steroids. If you take steroids you are going to grow no matter what you do at the gym. As a result, one guy is doing three sets per body part and another one is doing thirty. And the bottom line explanation given is "I go by how I feel."

Now you add to that personal trainers making up all kinds of ridiculous stuff in order to keep their clients entertained. Plus all the nonsense on social media. For someone who doesn't understand what is going on, it might really look like training is this journey to the mysterious land of unknown where everyone has to find their own path. No surprise that everybody at the gym is doing something completely different. You don't see such epidemic of variance in any other sport.

If you tell anyone just to stick to a few basic exercises and try to increase the weight by little every session, they are going to assume that you have not a slightest clue what you are talking about. "What about TRX face pulls or Bulgarian split squats?" Not to mention the fact that the moment you write it on a piece of paper it becomes a "cookie cutter" (aka not any good) program.

Individualization of training doesn't mean reinventing the wheel. It means fine tuning of a properly designed training program to optimize it for a specific person. This means that for the most part you should still follow the program. Unfortunately, that's asking too much for a lot of people. They would rather wander around the gym and make up stuff on the go. It's like people feel that their liberties are violated when you give them SPECIFIC training recommendations. "Individualization" is used as an excuse for such inability to follow a training plan. We get bored easily these days. Everything has to be fun.

"Individualization" of training is also being used to cover up unwillingness to research the topic a little. For some reason knowing how to train is considered a common sense. Therefore, if you need to research it, you must be stupid or something. Guys are especially "too cool for school" in this regard. It's almost like not knowing how to work out puts their masculinity in question. Just like no guy will ever openly say that he doesn't know what to do in the bedroom, he won't ever admit that he doesn't know what to do at the gym.

All the principles we discussed so far apply to every person at the gym. Unless you are working around injury or disability, no serious modification should be implemented at the beginner's level. You are just starting figuring out the training process. What is there to personalize? Do you think you just going to walk into a gym and come up with something nobody ever has thought of before?

If you think that you are the future Albert Einstein in the field of sport science, take into account that even he had many years of formal education before starting to propose his own theories. You should take the same approach. Learn the basics before exploiting your own creativity.

There are two main reasons to individualize training program. The first reason is to adjust it in accordance with your recovery capabilities (discussed in "energy budget" section). The second reason is to address weak points. For example, you might start doing a little extra work for your calves if you feel that they are your lagging muscle group (*priority principle*). Since none of these two reasons are a real concern in the initial stages of training, only intermediates should start experimenting with LIMITED modifications and only advanced athletes can fully rely on their own judgment while developing a training plan.

TERMINOLOGY

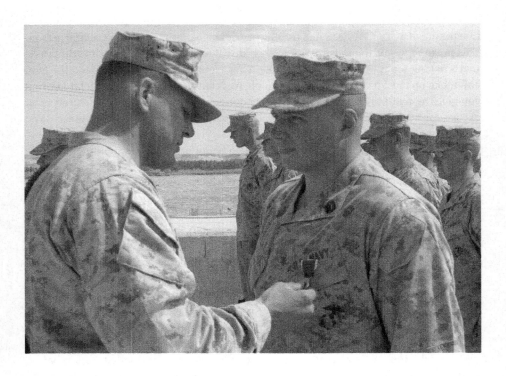

"Live for nothing or die for something."
– Quote from "Rambo"

Reps and sets

Lifting a load up and down one time is considered a repetition (*rep*). Performing a few repetitions in a row is called a set of repetitions (*set*). When training load is selected for a set it is usually estimated that the maximum number of reps it can be lifted (before fatiguing) will fall within a particular range. Desired number of repetitions per set will vary based on the goal. 1-6 reps are considered to be the best for strength development. 6-12 are the best for increasing the muscle size. 15 reps or higher are considered to be an endurance work. This is not to say that sets of 1 to 6 reps will not make you any bigger or doing 12 to 6 reps will not make you any stronger. Obviously, there is at least some overlap.

Sets are divided into warm up sets and work sets. The purpose of warm is to get you ready for the following work sets. Work sets are considered to be the sets in which you are handling the main training load (MTL) assigned for that session. The number of work sets per exercises is normally from 1 to 5. If the same load is being used for all work sets, they are referred to as *sets across*. If the load is increased from one work set to another, it is called a *pyramid*.

There are different ways to record sets and reps. For the purposes of this book the first number will be the sets and what follows after "x" will apply to reps. For example, 3x8-6 means three sets of eight to six reps. Unless otherwise specified, all work sets prescribed in this book are performed in sets across scheme.

The rest between sets will depend on the training mode of the session. During strength work long rest breaks (up to 5 minutes) are normally practiced. During hypertrophy sessions the rest breaks are kept shorter (around a minute) in order to maintain muscle "pump" from set to set. For the endurance training rest breaks are kept to 30 seconds or less and sometimes different exercises are rotated without any rest in between (*circuit training*).

The amount of rest between sets will also depend on the exercise itself. For example, you will need more rest between sets of squats than between sets of biceps curls. On occasion very heavy sets of deadlifts and squats might require rest breaks even longer than 5 minutes. In this case an effort must be made to stay warm and mentally focused.

Some other common gym terms related to reps and sets will be listed on the following page. Joe Weider is usually given the credit for systematizing these techniques. Their purpose is to shock muscles by taking them to the new level of exhaustion. It should be clear that absolutely NONE of these methods will be appropriate for beginners. Even the advanced athletes will have to apply them very sparingly as the risk of burnout is very high. Save these techniques for the last few sessions of Hypertrophy phases (NEVER Strength phases) and only for the stubborn body parts. There is no logical reason to hammer a muscle that still grows at a reasonable rate. Lee Haney said it best: "Exercise to stimulate, not to annihilate."

Partial reps – reps performed with less than full range of motion when due to fatigue an athlete can no longer complete a full repetition. For example, at the end of last set of pull-ups you could do a few reps with half or one third of full movement in order to push your muscles a little further.

Forced reps – reps performed with assistance of a training partner after an athlete can no longer continue the set on his own. For example, when the point of failure is reached in the bench press, training partner can provide just enough assistance to squeeze out one or two additional reps before terminating the set.

Rest-pause – the idea is very similar to the forced reps, but instead of getting help from a partner an athlete takes a short break at the end of the set and then continues with a few more reps. For example, once the point of total fatigue is reached in barbell rows, an athlete puts the barbell down for about 10-15 seconds and then picks it back up to complete additional two to three reps.

Drop-sets (aka *descending sets*) – once the point of exhaustion is achieved at the end of the set, the weight is immediately reduced so the athlete can continue with additional reps without getting any rest. For example, after doing as many repetitions as possible in lateral raises with 40 pound dumbbells, an athlete would grab a pair of 30s and continue with another 5-6 reps without getting any rest in between. This process could then be repeated one more time with 20s.

Supersets – two different exercises (usually for antagonistic muscle groups) performed without any rest in between. For example, after completing a set of biceps curls an athlete goes right to the set of pushdowns and only then gets to rest. This process is repeated in the same order as many times as was planned for the session. When the two exercises combined are targeting the same muscle group it is called *compound set*. These are usually arranged in such order that isolation movement precedes compound movement. For example, an athlete would "pre-exhaust" his quads with leg extensions and then go right into squats to really shock the muscle. Although it is possible to combine three (*trisets*) or even more exercises (*giant sets*) together, these techniques are typically out of the drug-free athlete's realm.

Warm up

Every exercise should be initiated with one to five warm-up sets. For the first warm-up set I usually recommend the same number of reps as is prescribed for the following work sets for that exercise, but with lighter weight. You can subtract one rep from each subsequent warm-up set as the weight increases. For example, if you are planning to deadlift 315lbs as your MTL for 5 sets of 5 reps, the warm-up could be the following:

> 135 for 5 reps
> 195 for 4 reps
> 255 for 3 reps

These are some of the general guidelines in regards to warm-up sets:

- The colder it is at the gym, the more extensive your warm-up might need to be.

- The more difficult exercises will generally require more warm-up than the easier ones. For example, you will probably need more warm-up sets for squats and deadlifts than for hammer curls or calf raises.

- The exercises that are earlier in your workout will normally require more sets than the later ones. For example, on the chest day in hypertrophy phase bench press might require three or more warm-up sets. Since your upper body is already warmed up after the bench press in the following incline dumbbell press you will probably need only one or two warm-up sets.

- The more advanced you get the more warm up you will probably require. It takes more time to get your body ready to deadlift 750 pounds than 75.

- Training sessions with lower reps will generally require more warm-up sets than training sessions with higher reps. Naturally when you are doing squats for 5x5 you will use a lot heavier weight than if you did 3x12-8. Therefore, the in the former training session you would need more time to warm up than in the latter.

- Straps and other grip aids should not be used during warm-up sets.

- Weightlifting belts should not be used during warm-up sets.

- Shortcutting warm up in attempt to save energy for work sets is NEVER a good idea.

!!! Warm-up sets are not included in the description of the training programs presented later in this book

Stretching

Most people confuse warm-up with stretching. They are not the same thing. To be able to stretch effectively you muscles have to be already warmed up, which makes the end of workout the best time for it. I would also suggest that you do some stretching combined with foam rolling on the off days. This is a great way to speed up the recovery and prevent injuries.

Learning how to properly stretch might not be as easy as it seems. Developing the ability to relax the muscle while stretching it will take some time. It is not "no pain, no gain" here. Static stretch positions are held for 30-60 seconds while slowly increasing the range of motion. Remember not to hold your breath while performing stretching.

Cardio

Cardio is layman's term and is generally being referred to a repetitive continuous activity involving large muscle groups. Detailed description of this topic would require another book to be written. The purpose of the discussion below is to give you a basic idea.

Cardio is usually being utilized to increase cardiovascular endurance (conditioning) or to lose fat. Conditioning is normally being trained by *intervals*: bouts of short intense effort (sprints, for example) separated by rest periods. The ratio of work/rest periods will be dictated by specific requirements of the particular sport. Most of the modern approaches also propose using targeted heart rate zones. However, unless you are an elite endurance athlete this is unnecessarily complicated.

For the purposes of burning fat continuous low intensity cardio is normally used. Fast pace walking is your best choice for two reasons. First, it is easier on the joints that are already being loaded by the heavy leg exercises. Second, it is less taxing and won't drain you as much as running. For this reason I would also not recommend high intensity interval training (HIIT) for the purposes of losing fat, something that became very popular lately. You might end up burning too much muscles mass in the process.

Only one of the programs presented here includes cardio. Before adding any amount of cardio to any other programs, make sure to review your priorities. Excessive cardio load will sap your energy rather quickly (remember the "energy budget" theory). Burning buckets of fat while adding pounds of muscle is a luxury of the steroid users. The rest of us have to take more cautious and patient approach.

EXERCISES

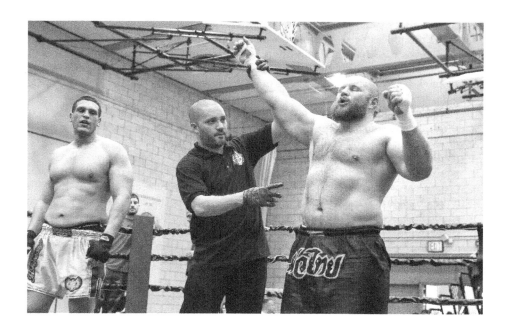

"You can't hit a target if you don't know what it is."

– Tony Robbins

Exercise descriptions presented here contain all the essential elements, but this is by no means an exhaustive list of all fine nuances. Such detailed description would go on for many pages for each exercise and could be overwhelming. As you get familiar with the basics presented here, make it a habit to do additional research. High mastery of exercise execution is a solid predictor of a long term success at the gym.

You will see many tips regarding safety. Do not dismiss them as trivia. The only way to achieve serious results in resistance training (assuming that proper methodology is utilized) is by sticking around long enough. Do not let an injury shorten your progress. *Careless attitude at the gym can turn something that is supposed to be beneficial for your health into a catastrophe.*

For example, I did not feel like bothering with safety collars during barbell exercises until I had plates rolling off on one side during squats. I did not think that using "thumbless" grip (thumbs are on the same side as the rest of the fingers) during bench press was that big of a deal until the bar slipped out of my hands and crushed into my chest. Luckily both of those instances happened during warm-up sets and did not cause a significant injury. Even more fortunate was the fact that, at least when it comes to the gym, I don't like to repeat the same mistake twice.

Another important, but often overlooked, aspect of training is that injuries do not happen only during the actual exercise execution. Awkward body mechanics while getting into starting position and returning the weight could put you at greater risk than the exercise itself.

Also, note that most exercises involving holding a weight in your hands will work forearm muscles to at least some extent. It is assumed and, therefore, not listed in the exercise descriptions. For that very reason no specialized exercises for forearms will be included in any of the programs. If your forearms are a lagging body part and you decide to include some direct work for them - proceed with caution. Forearms are taxed during most upper body exercises and any additional work must be carefully planned.

Back extension

Primary movers: spinal erectors.

Secondary movers: gluteus, hamstrings.

Starting position:

- Position the upper portion of your thighs firmly against the pads.
- Hook your heels under the roller pads.
- Keep your arms crossed on your chest.
- Tighten your lower back in slightly arched position.

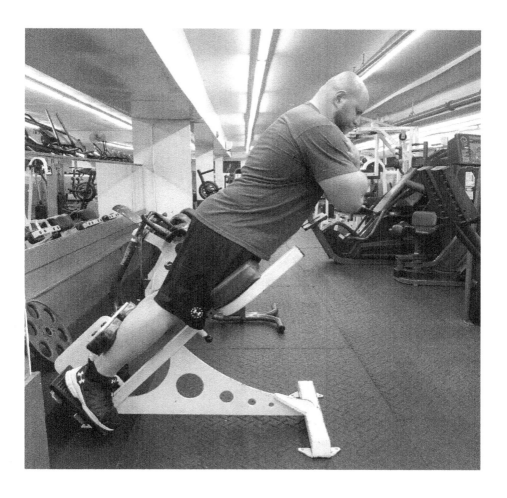

Movement:
- Lower you torso in controlled manner until it is almost perpendicular to the floor.
- Return to the starting position.

Common mistakes:
- Not going through full range of motion (ROM).
- Bouncing off from the bottom position.
- Excessive hyperextension at the top position.

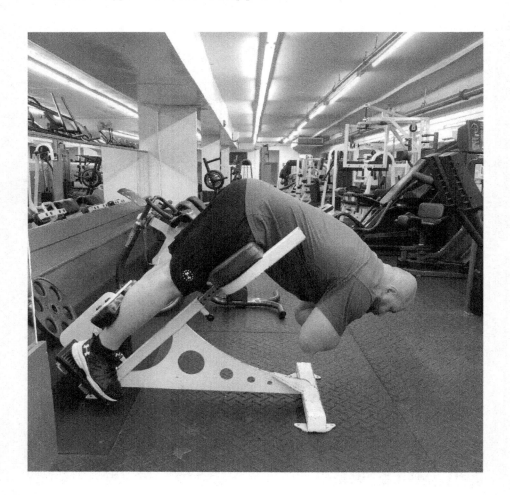

Back squat

Primary movers: quadriceps, gluteus, hamstrings.
Secondary movers: spinal erectors, adductors, calves.
Starting position:

- Find comfortable place for the bar on your upper traps (not on your neck).
- Place your hands palms facing forward over the bar slightly wider than your shoulder width (very wide grip makes it difficult to maintain tightness of the upper back needed to support the bar).
- Place your feet in line about shoulder width apart.
- Tighten your lower back in slightly arched position and bring your chest up.

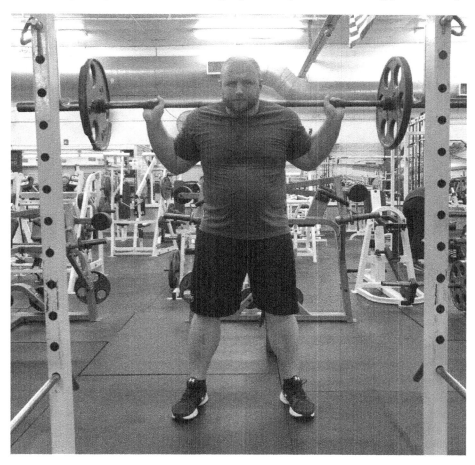

- Unrack the weight while keeping your back tight and take two steps back.
- Position your feet about shoulder width apart with toes pointing 20-30 degrees out.

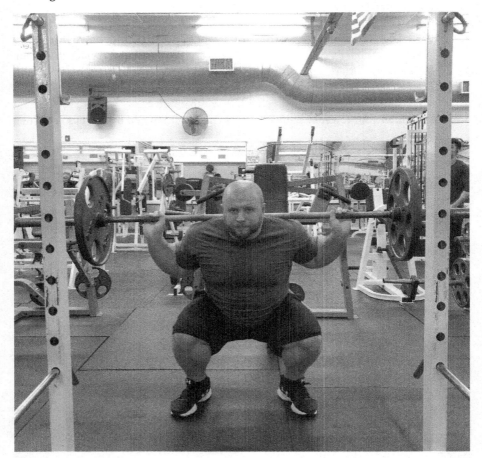

Movement:
- Simultaneously unlock your knees and hips and decent into position where your thighs are slightly below the parallel level with the floor.
- Do not exaggerate bounce at the bottom position.
- As you are coming up make sure that extension of hips and knees is happening at the same rate.
- Make sure the center of mass is over the middle of your feet the whole time.
- Maintain slight arch in your lower back at all time.

- Keep looking forward at the level slightly below your eye level.
- Make sure that your knees point in the same direction as your feet during both descent and ascent.
- Make sure to maintain tight torso until the bar is returned to the rack.
- Avoid any unnecessary rotation of the torso while moving the bar off and onto the rack.

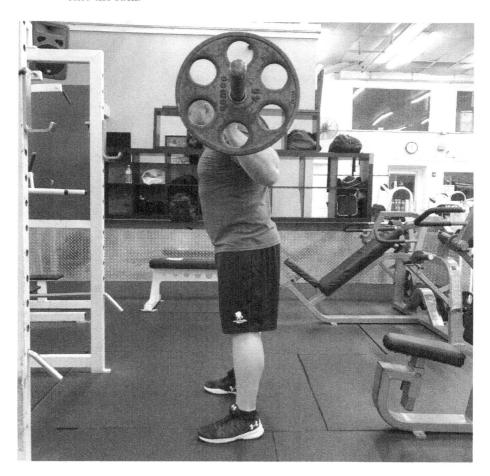

Common mistakes:
- Not descending deep enough (if consistent lack of depth is observed, it might be beneficial to perform squat with 1 second pause at the bottom during at least some of the warm-up sets).

- Excessive bending at the hips combined with lack of knee flexion (as in "Good Morning" exercise).
- Shifting center of the mass on heels or towards toes.
- Allowing the knees to move inwards on ascent/descent.
- Rounding your lower back.

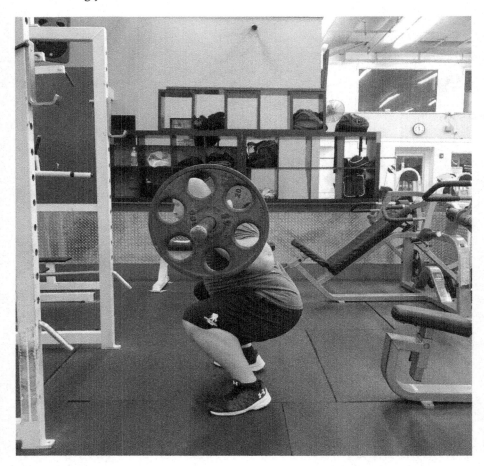

Alternative:
- Low bar position on the back might allow heavier loads to be used but will also shift some emphasis from quadriceps to hip extensors and lower back.

Caution:

- Even when a spotter is present, it is safer to perform squat inside power rack or with suspension straps.
- Weightlifting belt could be used for additional back support when very heavy loads are attempted.

Barbell bench press

Primary movers: pectorals.

Secondary movers: triceps, anterior deltoids.

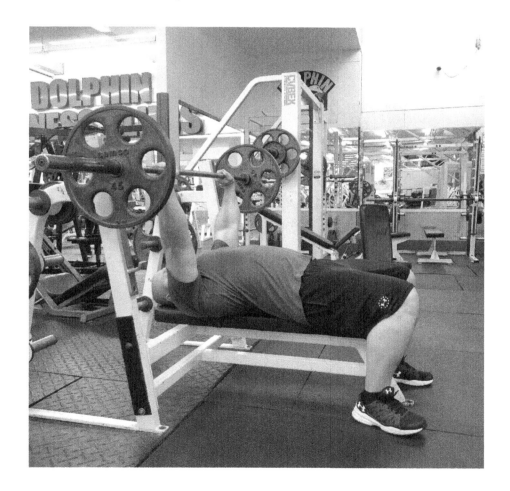

Starting position:

- Lie down on your back on flat bench.
- Slightly arch your lower back and bring your chest up.
- Squeeze your shoulder blades together.
- Place your feet flat on the floor with your knees bent at about 90 degrees.
- Grasp the bar with palms facing towards your legs.
- Select the grip width that will make your forearms parallel to each other (and perpendicular to the bar) at the point when the bar touches your chest.
- Position the bar in your hands between head line and life line of your palm with thumbs wrapped around.
- Unrack the bar and position it over your chest on extended arms.

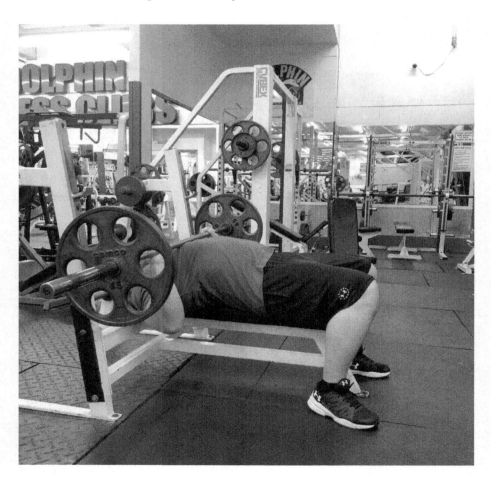

Movement:

- Lower the bar to your chest at about the level of your nipples (the movement will not be strictly vertical but rather a slight arc).
- Once you touch your chest, push it back up in the opposite direction until your arms are straight.
- Maintain elbows under the bar on both descent and ascent.
- Do not attempt to rack the bar until full elbow extension is attained.

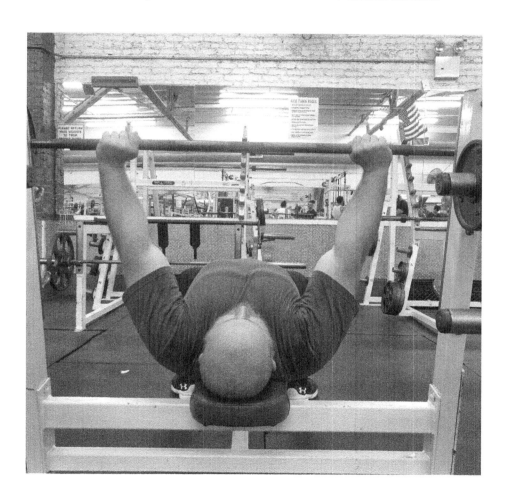

Common mistakes:

- Uneven descent/ascent of the bar.
- Allowing your buttocks to come off of the bench at any time.
- Lowering the bar too high on the chest (towards the neck)
- Bouncing the bar off of your chest.
- Not lowering the bar all the way to the chest.
- Not extending your elbows fully at the top of the movement (although hyperextension of elbows must also be avoided).
- Allowing your elbows to flare out excessively to the side.
- Excessive wrist extension during movement.
- Using thumbless grip.

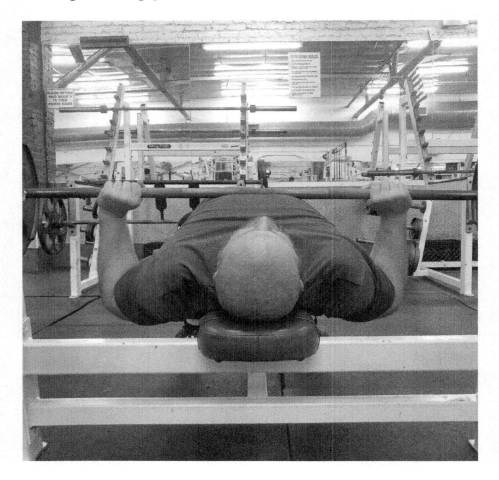

Alternative:

- Excessive arching of lower back reduces the distance the bar has to travel and allows to lift slightly heavier weight. Unless you are preparing for a powerlifting meet, however, this practice is counterproductive as *the business at the gym is not about making things easier.*

Caution:

- Presence of a spotter is a must when substantial load is being used.

Barbell bent-over row

Primary movers: lats.
Secondary movers: traps, posterior deltoids, biceps, spinal erectors.
Starting position:

- Bend your knees slightly and maintain that position throughout the exercise.
- Bend over at your hips while maintaining slight arch in your lower back.
- Grasp the bar with palms facing you, grip width slightly wider than your shoulders.
- Lift the weight off the floor with straight arms and position your torso at 20–30 degrees from parallel to the floor.

Movement:

- Pull the bar into the abdomen while squeezing your shoulder blades together.
- Avoid excessive upwards movement of the torso as you pull.
- Keep your elbows close to your body as you are moving the bar up.
- Once you touch your belly with the bar, return it back to starting position.
- Maintain slight arch in your lower back throughout.

Common mistakes:
- Rounding your lower back.
- Staying too upright during the exercise.
- Pulling the bar towards the chest instead of abdomen.
- Swinging the weight up with the help from the hips.
- Not going through full ROM (usually means that the weight is too heavy).

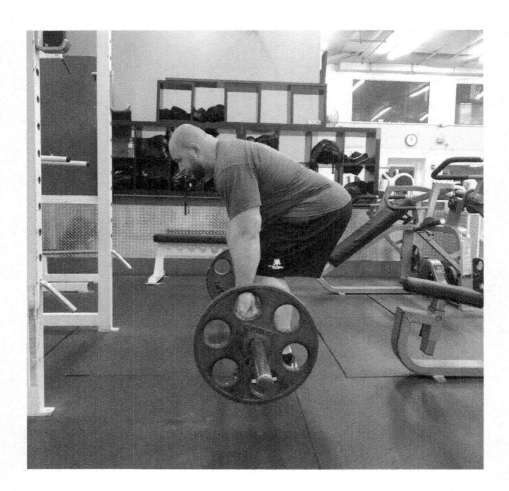

Alternative:

- If significant load is being used (usually in Strength phases), the bar can be returned to the floor after each rep.

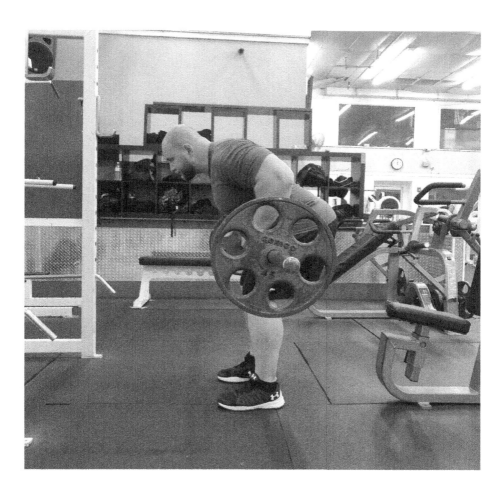

Caution:

- Weightlifting belt could be used for additional back support when very heavy loads are attempted.

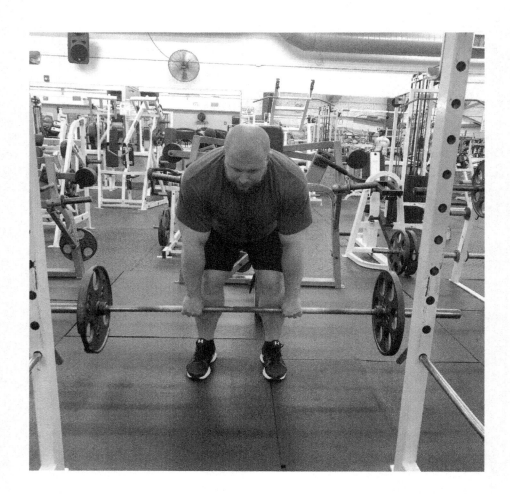

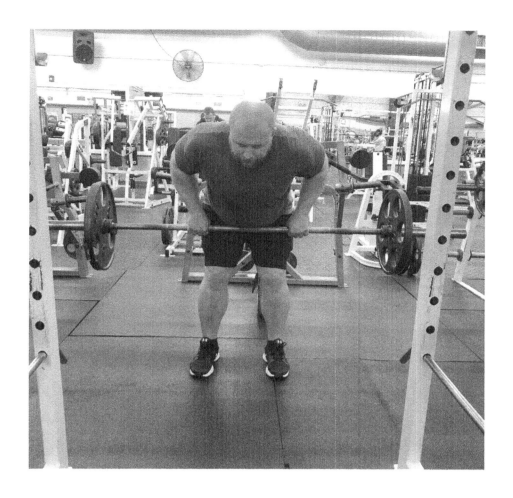

Barbell biceps curl

Primary movers: biceps.
Secondary movers: brachialis, brachioradialis.
Starting position:

- Stand in front of the bar with your feet shoulder width apart.
- Unlock your knees and tighten your lower back in slightly arched position.
- Grasp a bar with shoulder width grip with palms facing away.

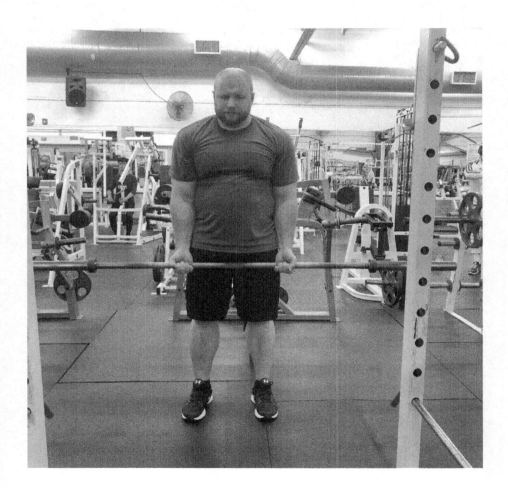

Movement:
- Bend your elbows without any significant movement at any other body parts.
- Squeeze your biceps at the top and bring the bar down under control.
- Keep your elbows tucked in against your rib cage.

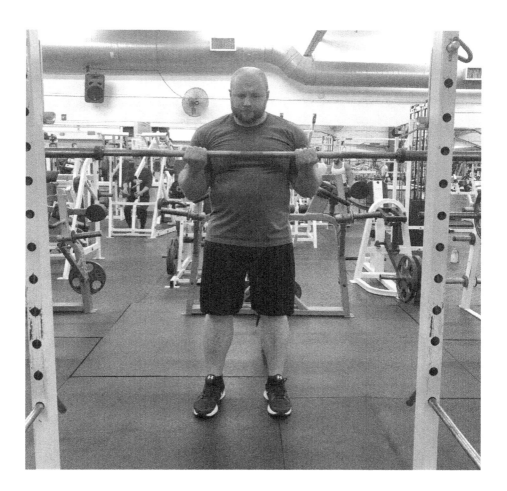

Common mistakes:

- Excessive wrist movement during descent/ascent.
- Swinging the weight up with upper body.
- Allowing the elbows to flare out to the sides.
- Excessive shoulder flexion on the upward movement.
- Not going through full ROM (usually lacking a full elbow extension at the bottom).

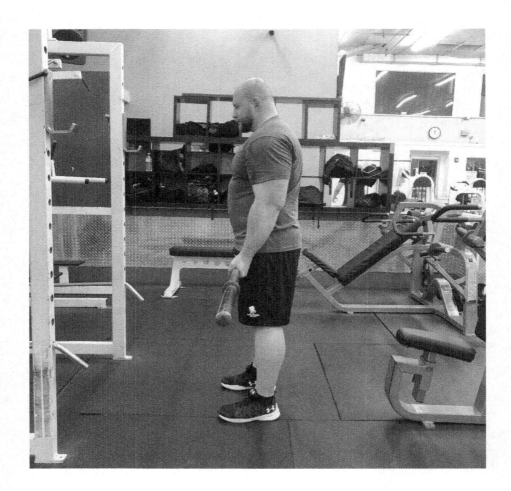

Alternative:

- EZ–bar can be used if straight bar causes wrist pain.

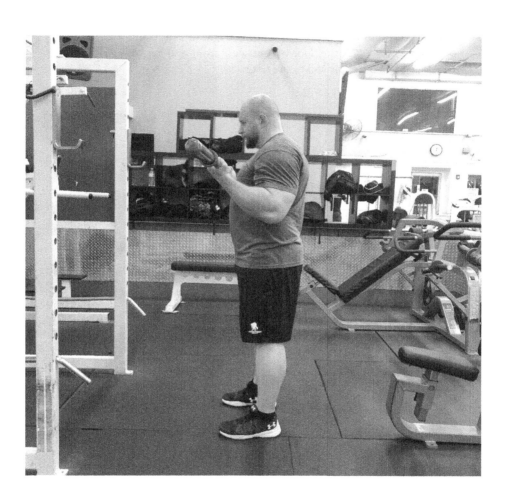

Bent-over dumbbell raise

Primary movers: posterior deltoids.

Secondary movers: traps, spinal erectors.

Starting position:

- Bend your knees slightly and maintain that position throughout the exercise.
- Bend over at your hips while maintaining slight arch in your lower back.
- Lift the dumbbells off the floor with straight arms and position your torso at 20-30 degrees from parallel to the floor.

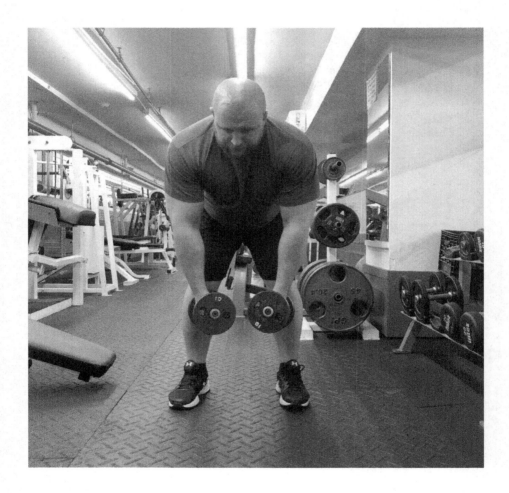

Movement:
- With your elbows slightly bent, raise your arms to the sides as high as you can.
- Squeeze your shoulder blades together at the top and return to the starting position.

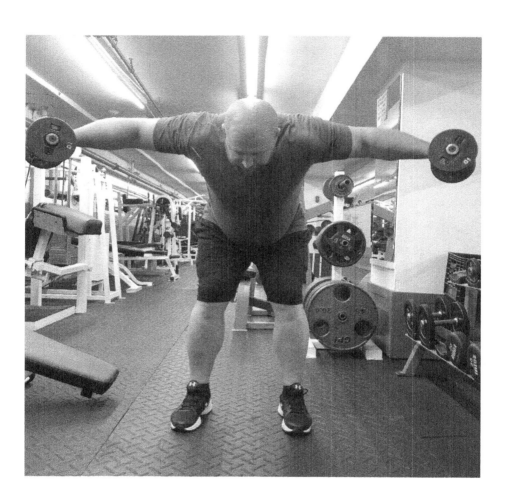

Common mistakes:

- Rounding your lower back.
- Staying too upright during the exercise.
- Swinging the weight up with the help from the hips.
- Excessive bending of the elbows (which turns exercise into "Dumbbell Row").
- Not going through full ROM (usually means that the weight is too heavy).

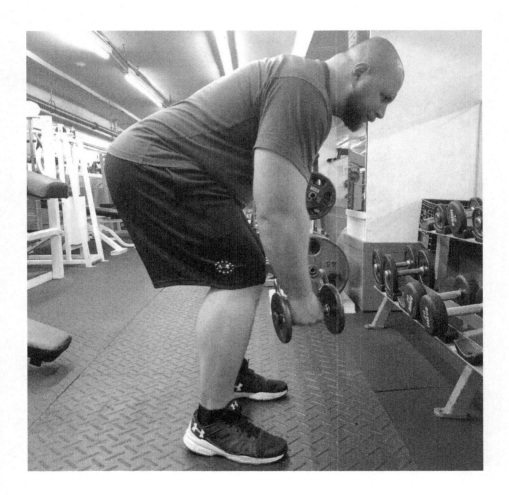

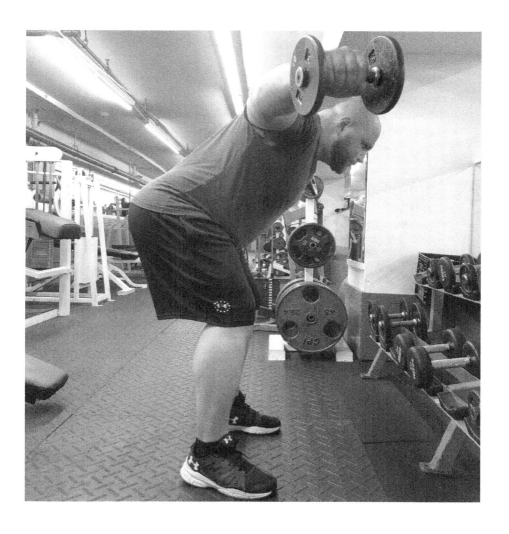

Chin-up

Primary movers: lats, biceps.

Secondary movers: posterior deltoids.

Starting position:

- Position your hands on the bar with shoulder width grip, palms facing you.
- Hang off of the bar on straight arms and allow your shoulder blades to come slightly out and up.

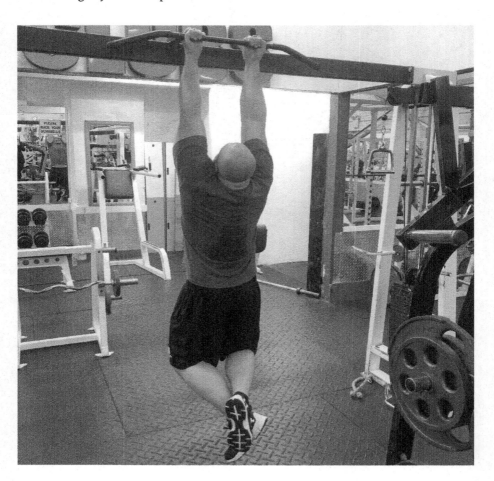

Movement:
- Pull yourself up while bringing your chest up.
- Try to touch the bar with your chest while squeezing your shoulder blades together.
- Lower yourself under control back to starting position.

Common mistakes:
- Not going through full ROM.
- Creating momentum by swinging your legs.

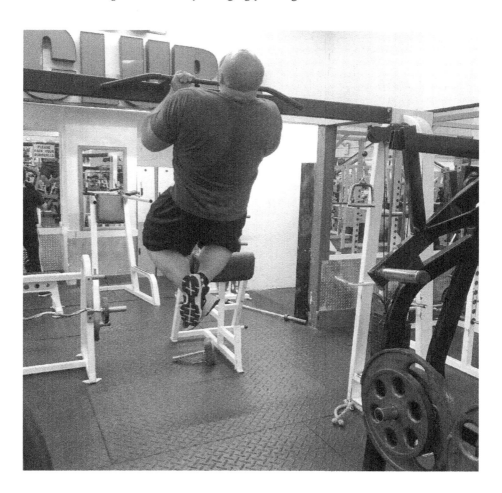

Close grip barbell bench press

Primary movers: triceps.

Secondary movers: chest, anterior deltoids.

Starting position:

- Lie down on your back on flat bench.
- Slightly arch your lower back and bring your chest up.
- Squeeze your shoulder blades together.
- Place your feet flat on the floor with your knees bent at about 90 degrees.
- Grasp the bar shoulder width or slightly narrower with palms facing towards your legs.

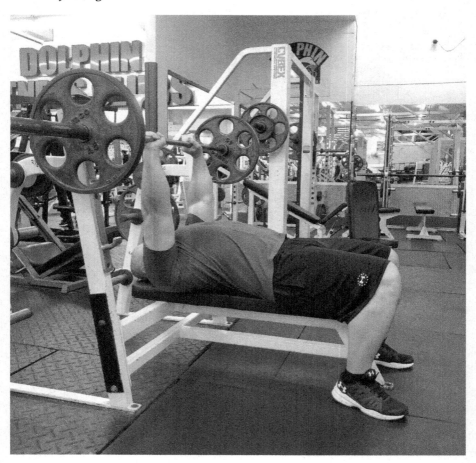

- Position the bar in your hands between head line and life line of your palm with thumbs wrapped around.
- Unrack the bar and position it over your chest on extended arms.

Movement:
- Lower the bar to your chest slightly below the level of your nipples.
- Once you touch your chest, push it back up in the opposite direction until your arms are straight.
- Keep your elbows tucked in against your rib cage in the lower portion of the movement.
- Do not attempt to rack the bar until full elbow extension is attained.

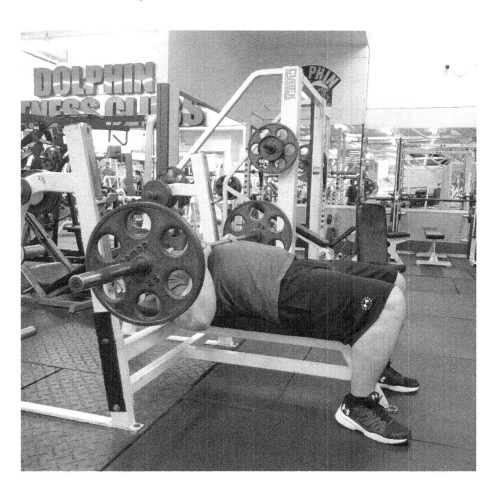

Common mistakes:

- Lowering the bar too high on the chest (towards the neck)
- Uneven descent/ascent of the bar.
- Allowing your buttocks to come off of the bench at any time.
- Bouncing the bar off of your chest.
- Allowing your elbows to flare out excessively to the side.
- Not lowering the bar all the way to the chest.
- Not extending your elbows fully at the top of the movement (although hyperextension of elbows must also be avoided).
- Excessive wrist movement during descent/ascent.
- Using thumbless grip.

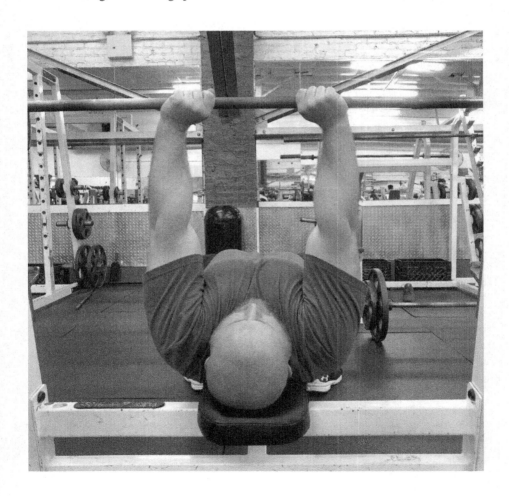

Caution:
- Presence of a spotter is a must when substantial load is being used.
- Using grip width much narrower than shoulder width puts a lot of additional stress on the wrists.

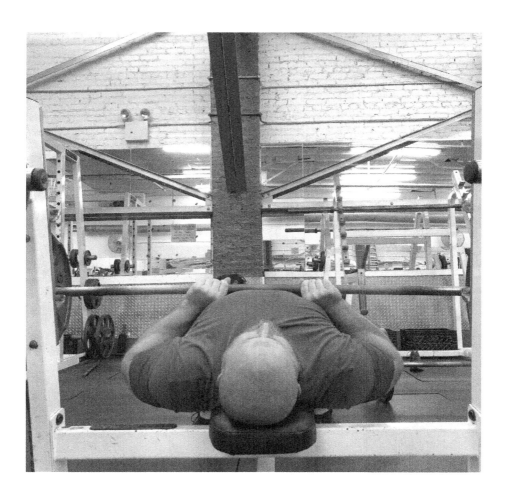

Deadlift

Primary movers: spinal erectors, gluteus, hamstrings, quadriceps.

Secondary movers: lats, traps.

Starting position:

- Place your feet shoulder width or slightly narrower with your toes pointing forward (or slightly out).
- Before you bend over to grasp the bar your shins should be about an inch away from it.
- Tighten your lower back in slightly arched position and maintain it throughout the exercise.

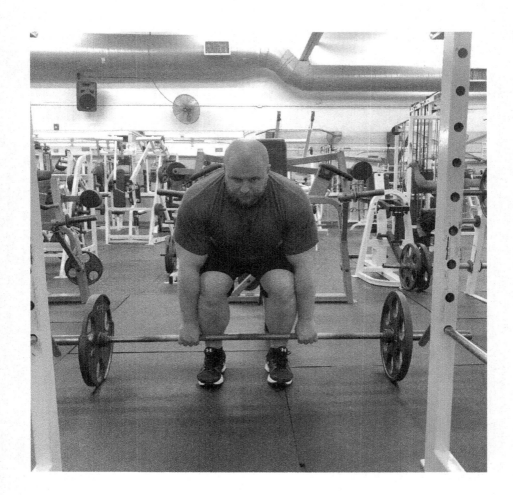

- Squat down to grasp the bar while flexing slightly more at the hips and slightly less at your knees when compared to the back squat.
- Grasp the bar with the grip right outside of your legs with palms facing you.
- Keep your chest up and your shoulders slightly in front of the bar.
- Look straight forward.

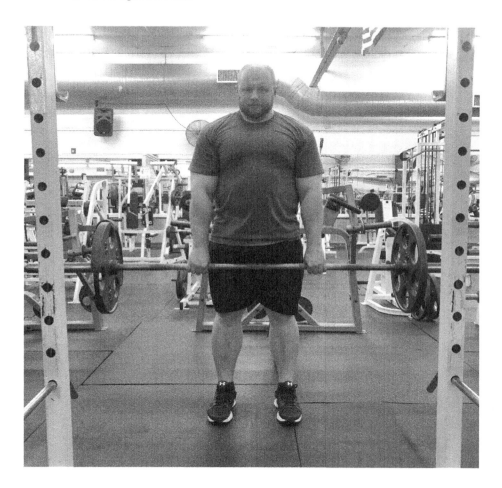

Movement:
- Stand up with the bar held in completely straight arms.
- Make sure the bar stays in contact with your legs the whole time.
- Once the fully upright position is attained, lower the bar back on the floor.

- Make sure that your knees point in the same direction as your feet during both descent and ascent.
- Do not try to bounce the weight off the floor for the following rep.

Common mistakes:
- Rounding your lower back.
- Allowing the knees to move inwards on ascent/descent.
- Allowing the bar to drift away from the front of the legs (usually the result of premature straightening of the legs in the beginning of movement).
- Excessive hyperextension at the top.
- Bending of the elbows.

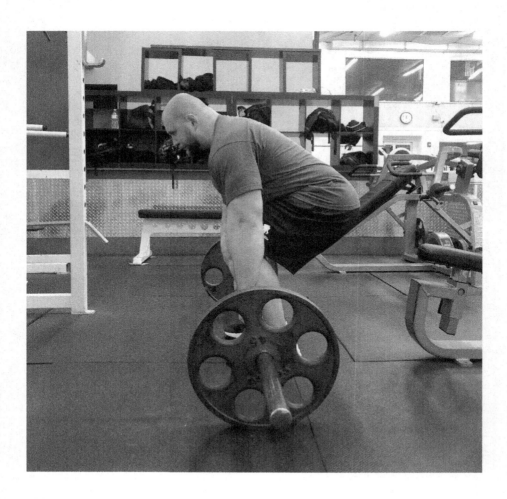

Caution:

- Even though *alternated grip* (one hand supinated, one hand pronated) is often utilized, its use presents an inherent danger. Unless you are planning to compete in powerlifting contest, use straps when the grip becomes a weak point of the lift.
- Weightlifting belt could be used for additional back support when very heavy loads are attempted

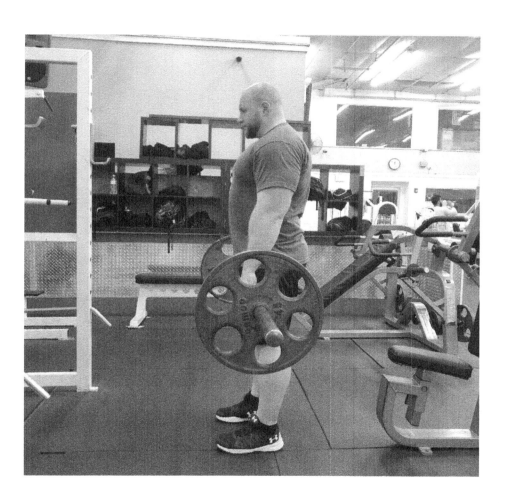

Dip

Primary movers: lower pectorals, triceps.

Secondary movers: anterior deltoids.

Starting position:

- Position yourself between parallel bars while supported on the straight arms.

Movement:

- Lower yourself while slightly tilting your torso forward.
- Once a good pectoral stretch is attained, bring yourself back to the starting position.

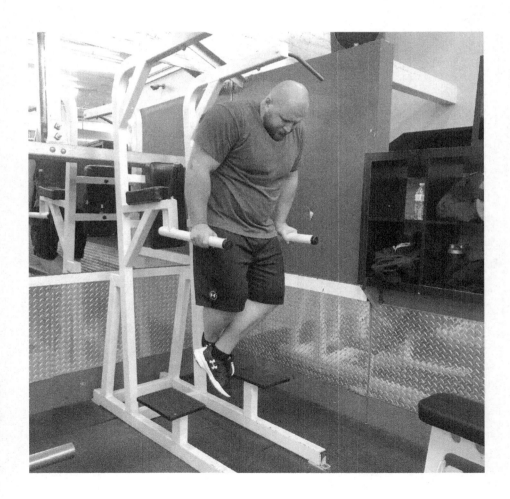

Common mistakes:
- Not going through full ROM.
- Going too low on the descent (tough on shoulder joints).
- Allowing your elbows to flare out excessively to the side.
- Bouncing off from the bottom position.
- Creating momentum by swinging your legs.

Caution:
- Modifying torso positions to emphasize different muscles could also increase stress on certain joints.

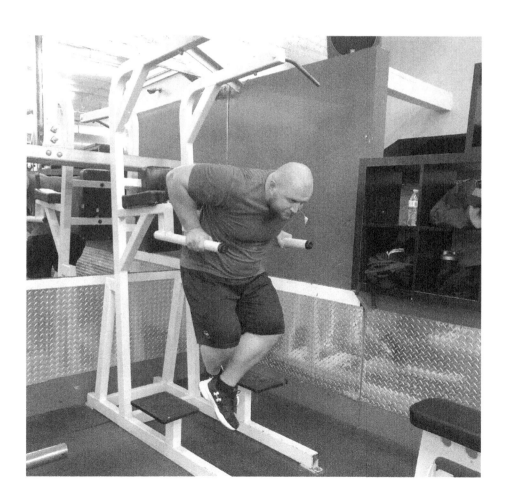

Dumbbell bench press

Primary movers: pectorals.
Secondary movers: anterior deltoids, triceps.

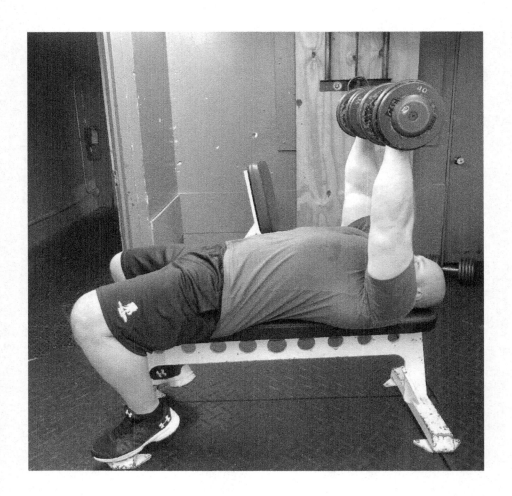

Starting position:
- Lie down on your back on flat bench.
- Slightly arch your lower back and bring your chest up.
- Squeeze your shoulder blades together.
- Position a pair of dumbbells over your chest on straight arms with palms facing towards your legs (help of a spotter might be needed to get into starting position).

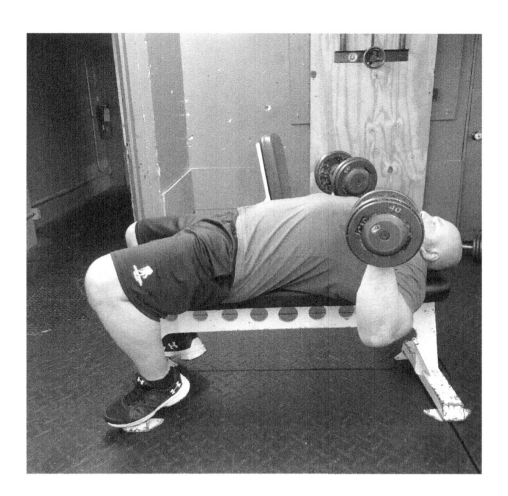

Movement:

- Lower dumbbells to your sides in wide arc while keeping your forearms parallel to each other.
- Once good pectoral stretch is attained, push the dumbbells up and together until the arms are straight.

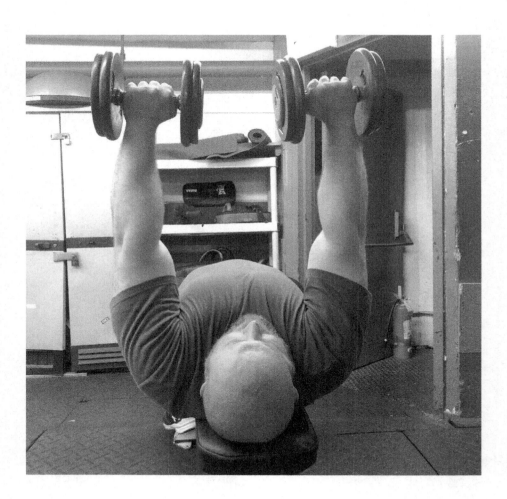

Common mistakes:
- Allowing the buttocks to come off the bench.
- Not going through full ROM.

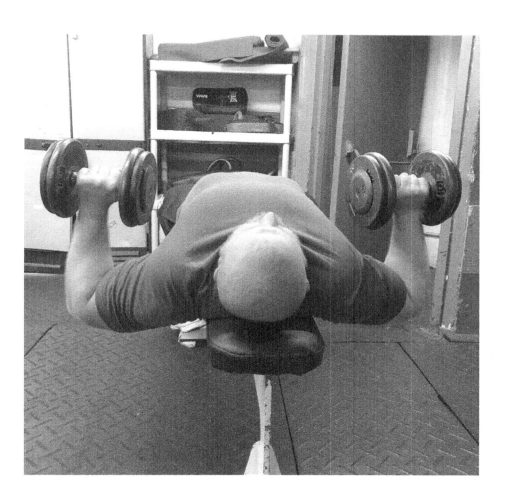

Dumbbell hammer curl

Primary movers: brachialis, biceps, brachioradialis.

Starting position:

- Stand with your feet shoulder width apart.
- Position dumbbells at your sides with palms facing each other.

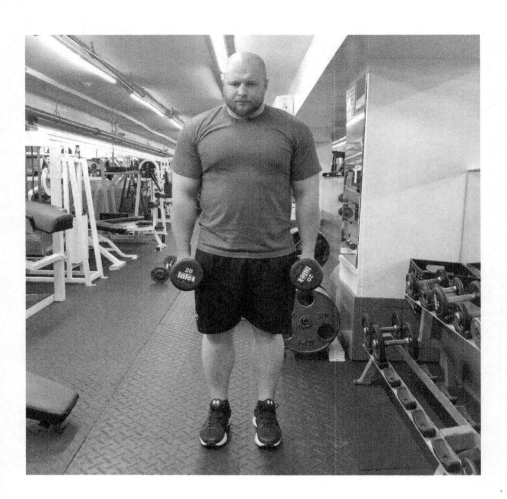

Active movement:
- Bend your elbows without any significant movement at any other body parts.
- Squeeze your biceps at the top and bring the dumbbells down under control.
- Keep your elbows tucked in against your rib cage.

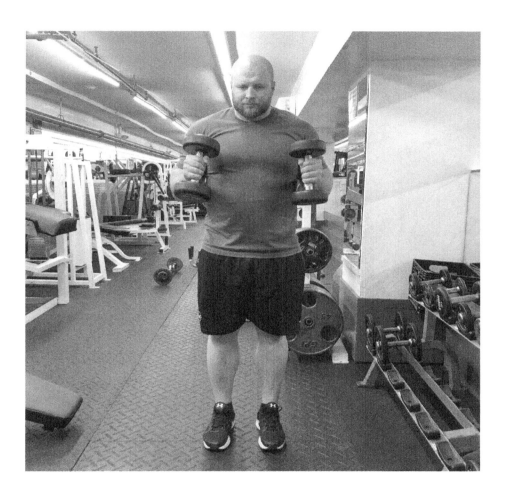

Common mistakes:

- Swinging the weight up with upper body.
- Allowing the elbows to flare out to the sides.
- Excessive shoulder flexion on the upward movement.
- Not going through full ROM (usually lacking a full elbow extension at the bottom).

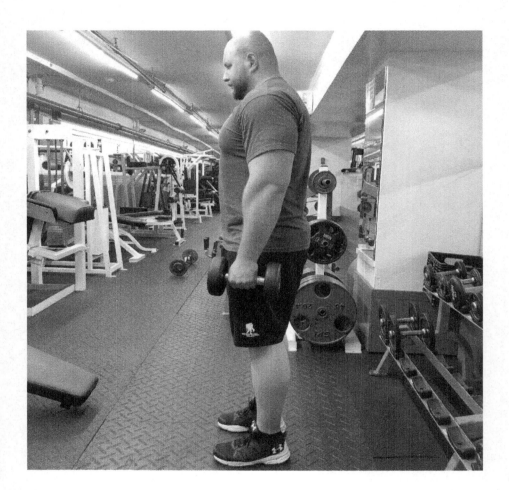

Alternative:
- Exercise can be performed in alternating manner: as one dumbbell comes down, another one comes up.

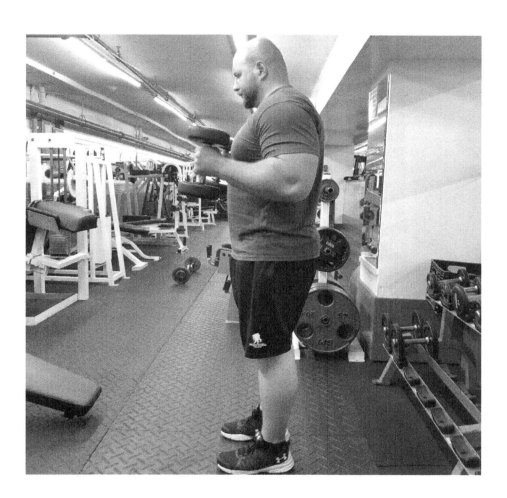

Dumbbell shoulder press

Primary movers: anterior and lateral deltoids.

Secondary movers: triceps, traps.

Starting position:

- Sit on the chair with back support (as shown) or stand with your feet shoulder width apart.
- Keep your chest high.
- Position dumbbells on the sides of your shoulders at about chin level.
- Palms facing forward but could also be slightly turned in.

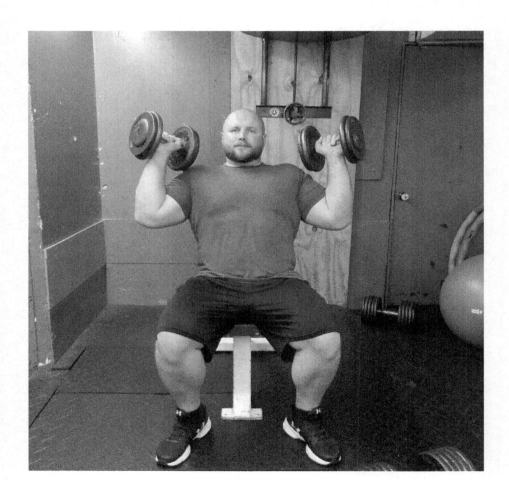

Movement:
- Press the dumbbells up and together over your head until arms are straight.
- Return dumbbells into starting position.

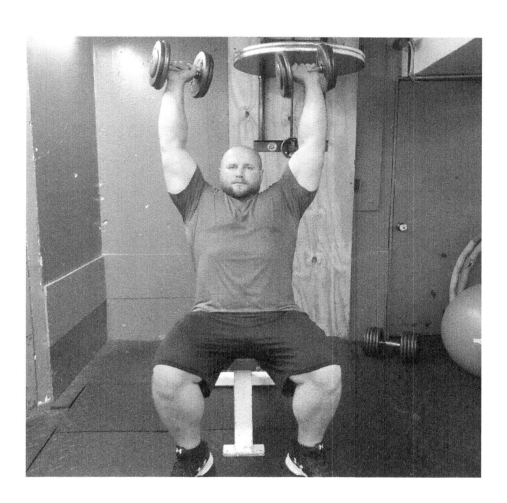

Common mistakes:
- Not going through the full ROM.
- Pressing the dumbbells forward instead of over your head.
- Not maintaining elbows directly under the dumbbells.

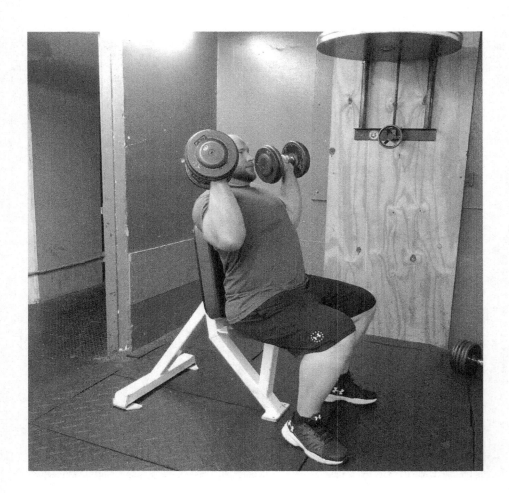

Alternative:

- Seated position usually allows you to use slightly heavier weights, however, might require help of a spotter with getting dumbbells into starting position.

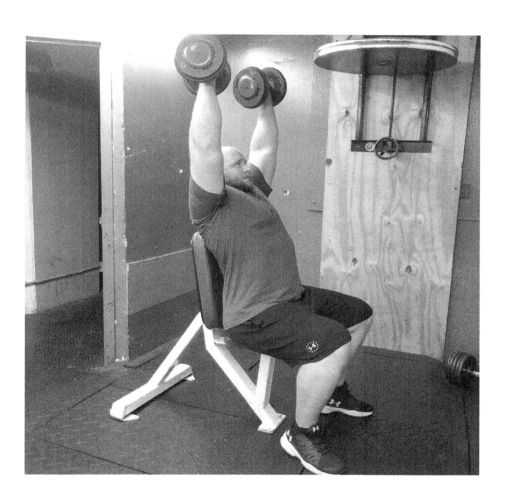

Dumbbell shrug

Primary movers: traps.

Starting position:

- Stand in front of the bar with your feet shoulder width apart.
- Unlock your knees and tighten your lower back in slightly arched position.
- Position dumbbells at your sides with palms facing each other.

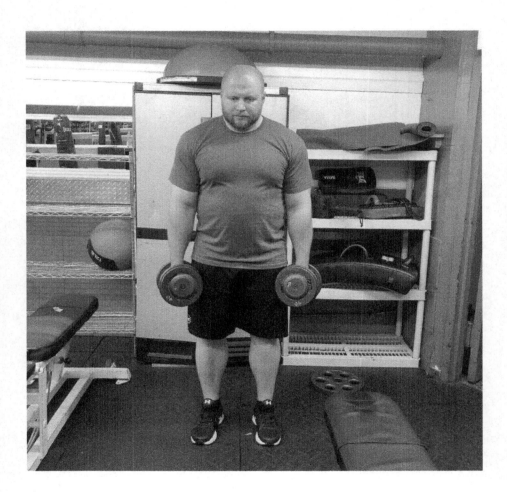

Active movement:
- Shrug your shoulders as high up as you can while simultaneously tilting your head slightly forward.
- Return dumbbells to the starting position.

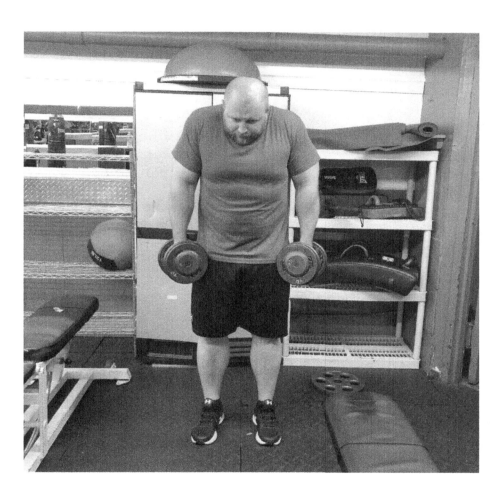

Common mistakes:
- Bending your elbows excessively on the upward movement.
- Not going through full ROM (usually means that the weight is too heavy).
- Swinging the weight up by involving your legs.

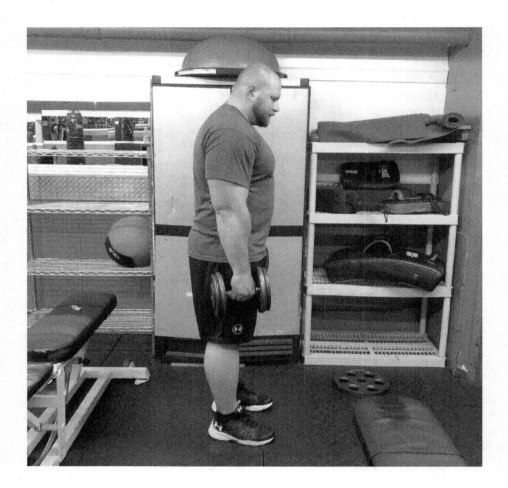

Alternative:

- If the gym doesn't have dumbbells that are heavy enough, perform "Barbell Shrugs" instead.

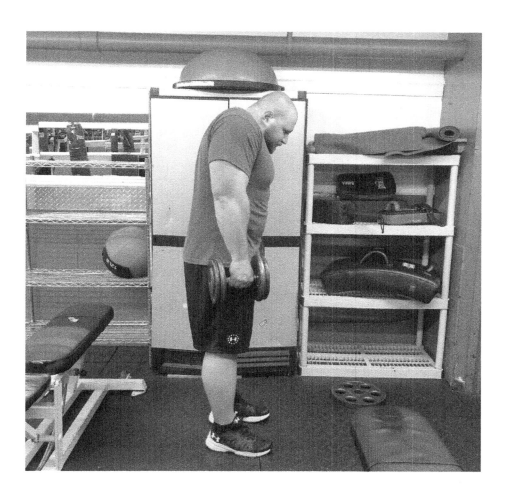

Front squat

Primary movers: quadriceps, gluteus.

Secondary movers: hamstrings, adductors, spinal erectors, calves.

Starting position:

- Find comfortable place for the bar on your chest just behind anterior deltoids.
- Place your hands palms facing forward under the bar slightly wider than your shoulder width and rotate your elbows up.
- Place your feet about shoulder width apart.
- Tighten your lower back in slightly arched position and bring your chest up.
- Unrack the weigh while keeping your back tight and take two steps back.
- Position your feet about shoulder width apart with toes pointing slightly out.

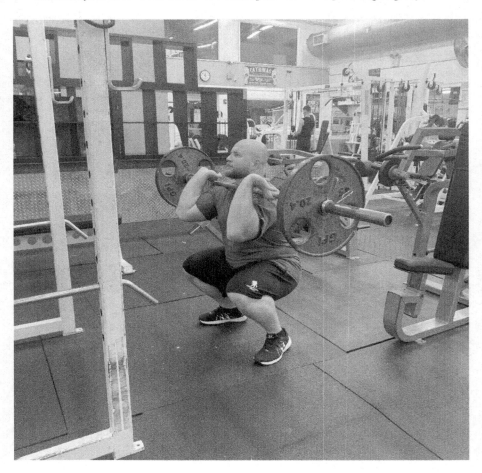

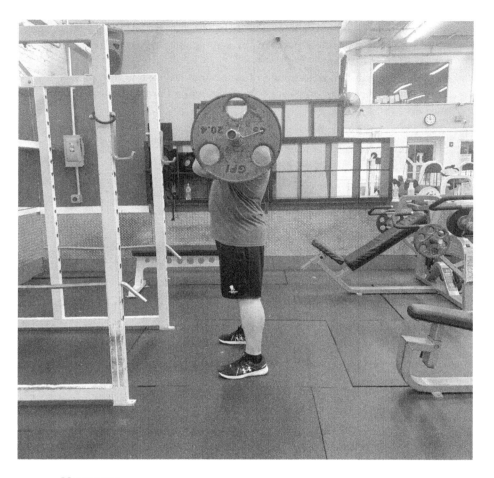

Movement:
- While maintaining torso almost vertical, unlock your knees and descend into position where your thighs are slightly below the parallel level with the floor.
- Allow your knees to move past your toes further forward than they would in back squat (difficulty in doing so might be an indication of insufficient ankle mobility).
- Do not exaggerate bounce at the bottom position.
- As you coming up make sure to maintain your torso vertical and your elbows pointing forward.
- Make sure the center of mass is over the middle of your feet the whole time.
- Maintain slight arch in your lower back at all time.

- Keep looking forward at the level slightly below your eye level.
- Make sure that your knees point in the same direction as your feet during both descent and ascent.
- Make sure to maintain tight torso until the bar is returned to the rack.
- Avoid any unnecessary rotation of the torso while moving the bar off and onto the rack.

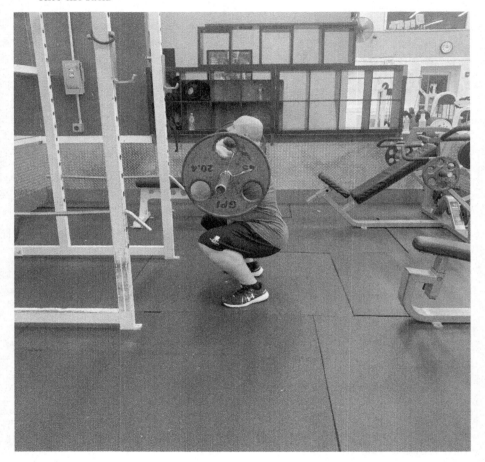

Common mistakes:
- Not descending deep enough.
- Failure to maintain upright torso (might result falling of the bar off of the chest).
- Shifting center of the mass on heels or towards toes.

- Allowing the knees to move inwards on ascent/descent.

Alternative:

- If due to lack of flexibility proper elbow position cannot be attained, temporarily use the grip with arms crossed on your chest (shown below).

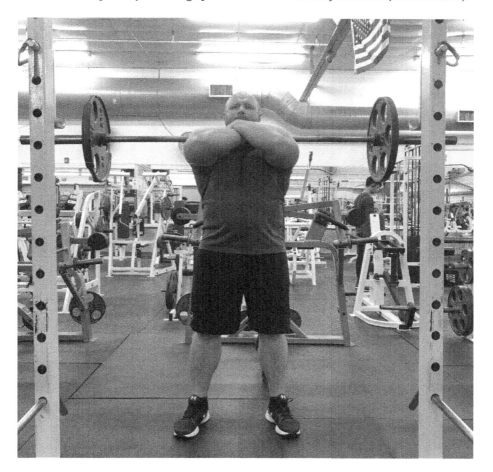

Caution:
- Pushing the bar too high into the neck might result a syncopal episode.
- An athlete must be prepared to jump from under the bar if the lift is missed.
- Weightlifting belt could be used for additional back support when very heavy loads are attempted.

Goblet squat

Primary movers: quadriceps, gluteus.

Secondary movers: hamstrings, adductors, spinal erectors, calves.

Starting position:

- Place your feet in line about shoulder width apart (perhaps slightly wider than in back squat and with your feet turned slightly more out).
- Tighten your lower back in slightly arched position and bring your chest up.
- Hold a dumbbell with two hands by your chest at the level slightly below your chin.

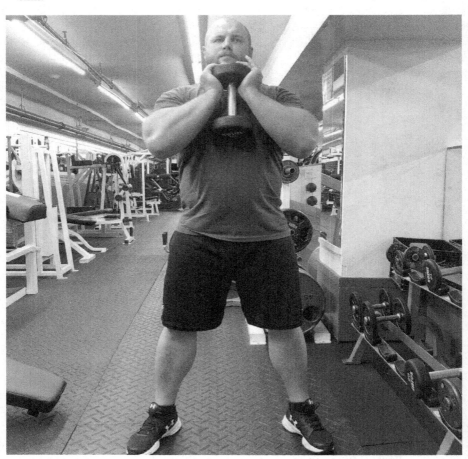

Movement:

- Unlock your knees and descend into position where your thighs are slightly below the parallel level with the floor while maintaining torso almost vertical.
- Do not exaggerate bounce at the bottom position.
- As you coming up make sure to maintain your torso upright.
- Make sure the center of mass is over the middle of your feet the whole time.
- Maintain slight arch in your lower back at all time.
- Keep looking forward at the level slightly below your eye level.
- Make sure that your knees point in the same direction as your feet during both descent and ascent.

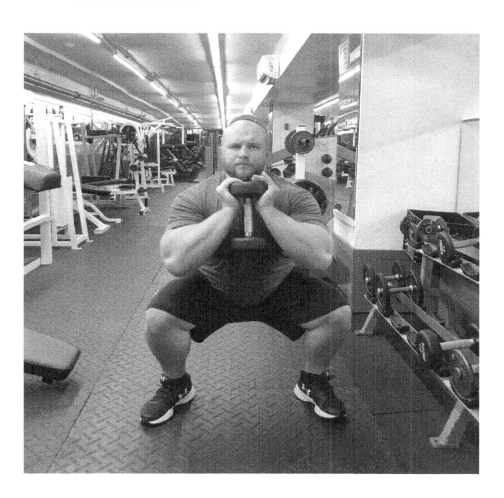

Common mistakes:
- Not descending deep enough.
- Rounding your lower back.
- Failure to maintain upright torso (in this case you might feel that your weight is shifting to the front of your feet).
- Allowing the knees to move inwards on ascent/descent.
- Bouncing from the bottom of the squat.

Hang power clean

Primary movers: quadriceps, gluteus, spinal erectors, hamstrings.
Secondary movers: traps, deltoids, calves.

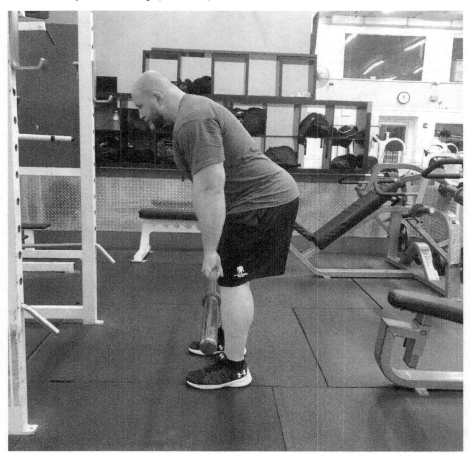

Starting position:

- Stand in front of the bar with your feet in position similar to that of the deadlift.
- Grasp the bar with the grip width similar to the one you use for front squat (it is easier to learn this move if at least some proficiency in front squat is achieved).
- Use of *hook grip* (thumbs wrapped around by the rest of the fingers) is generally recommended.
- Tighten your lower back in slightly arched position.
- The bar should be touching your legs just above your knee caps.
- At the starting position your shoulders should be slightly more forward than they would be at this height in deadlift.

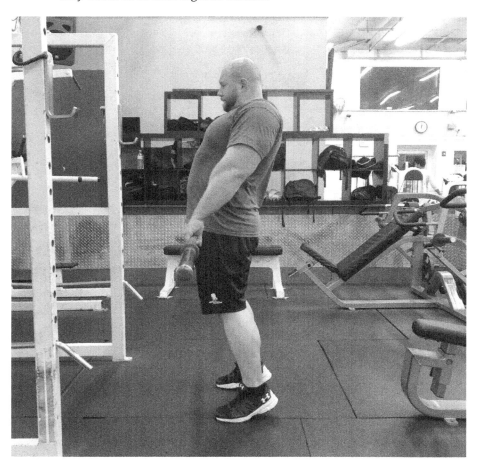

Movement:

- While keeping your arms straight, explosively pull the bar up by simultaneously extending your hips and your knees (similarly to how you would do if you were trying to jump straight up).
- As the bar moving up by the momentum created by the pull, drop down to about a quarter of the front squat position.
- Catch the bar on your chest with your elbows high.
- Stand up with the bar secured on your chest (as in starting position of the front squat).
- Drop the bar off of your chest and catch it by the lower portion of your thighs.
- You might have to reset your feet between each rep.

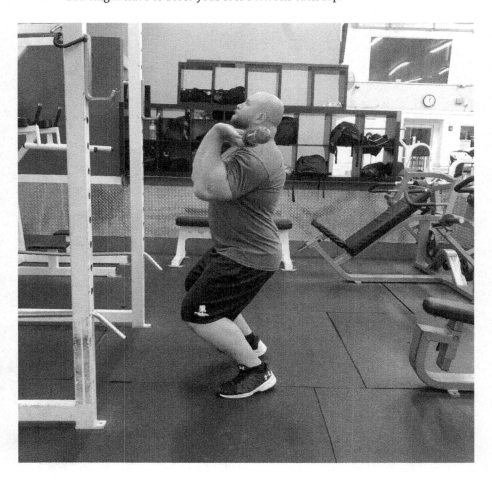

Common mistakes:
- Performing this exercise as ballistic reverse grip biceps curl.
- Catching the bar on your hands instead of the chest.
- Overemphasized arm pull (as in "Upright Row" exercise).
- Allowing the knees to move inwards on ascent/descent.
- Rounding your lower back.
- Trying to lower the bar slowly.

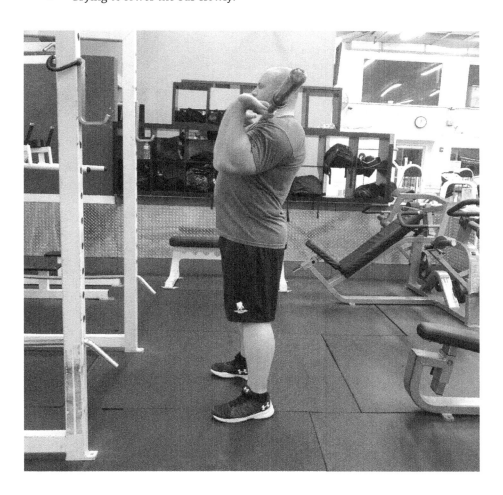

Caution:
- Catching the bar too high on the chest might result a syncope episode.
- An athlete must be prepared to jump away from the bar if the lift is missed.
- Weightlifting belt could be used for additional back support when very heavy loads are attempted.

Incline dumbbell press

Primary movers: upper pectorals.
Secondary movers: anterior deltoids, triceps.

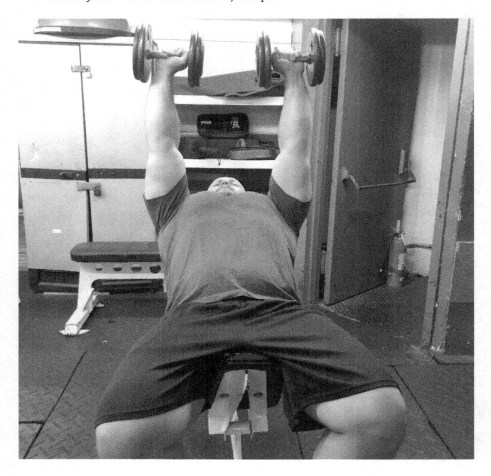

Starting position:
- Lie down on incline bench (about 30–40 degrees from horizontal).
- Bring your chest up and squeeze your shoulder blades together.
- Position a pair of dumbbells over your face on straight arms with palms facing towards your legs (help of a spotter might be needed to get into starting position).

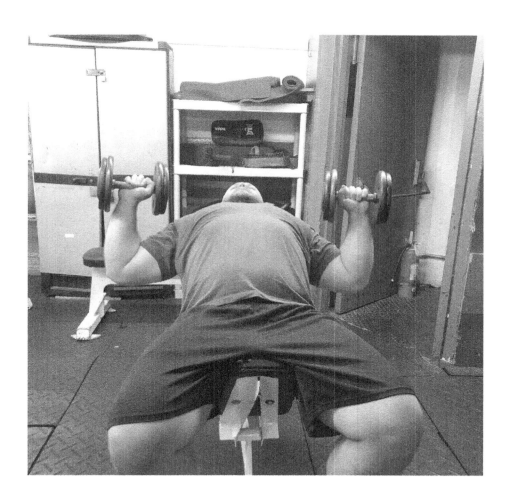

Movement:
- Lower dumbbells to your sides in wide arc while keeping your forearms parallel to each other.
- Once good pectoral stretch is attained, push the dumbbells up and together until the arms are straight.

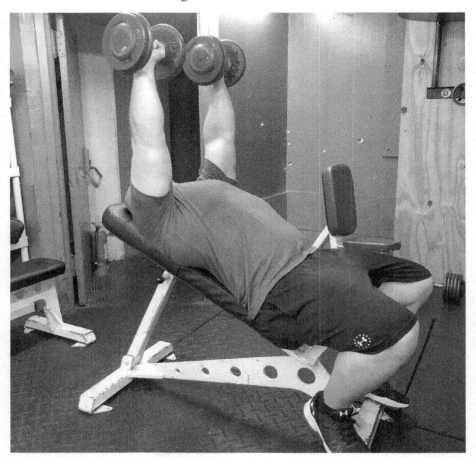

Common mistakes:
- Allowing the buttocks to come off the bench.
- Not going through full ROM.

Alternative:

- "Incline Barbell Press" can be used instead if the gym doesn't have heavy enough dumbbells.

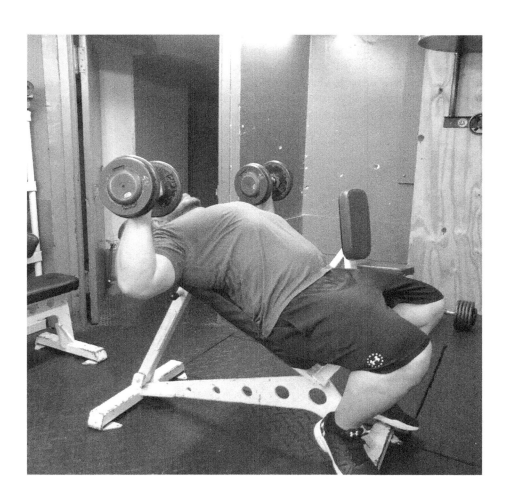

Incline sit-up

Primary movers: abdominals.

Secondary movers: hip flexors.

Starting position:

- Hook your feet under the roller pads.
- Lie down on the incline bench with your head down (the higher your legs in relation to the head, the more difficult the exercise will be).
- Tuck your chin down to your chest.
- Cross your arms on your chest with your fingers touching your shoulders (unless you are holding a plate on your chest).

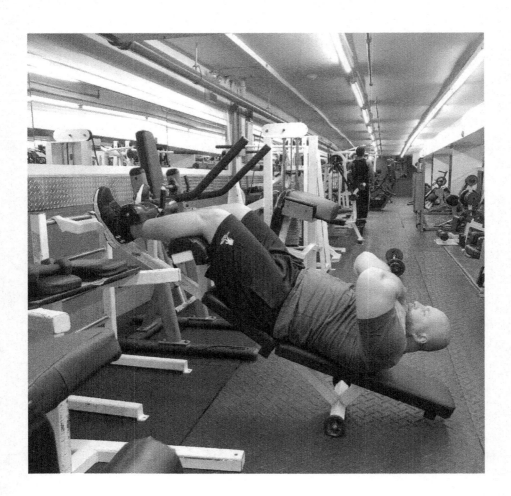

Movement:
- Curl your torso up and touch the lower portions of your thighs with your elbows.
- Return to the starting position.

Common mistakes:
- Not keeping your hands in contact with the shoulders (if you are holding a plate, keep it close to your chin).
- Pulling on your head during ascent.
- Performing the ascent in ballistic fashion.
- Keeping the torso very rigid (will make hip flexors do most of the work).

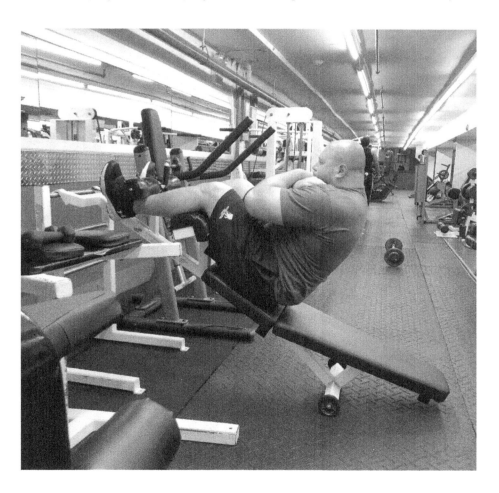

Alternative:

- Out of shape beginners might need to start with "Crunches" (shown below) and switch to sit-ups a few months later.

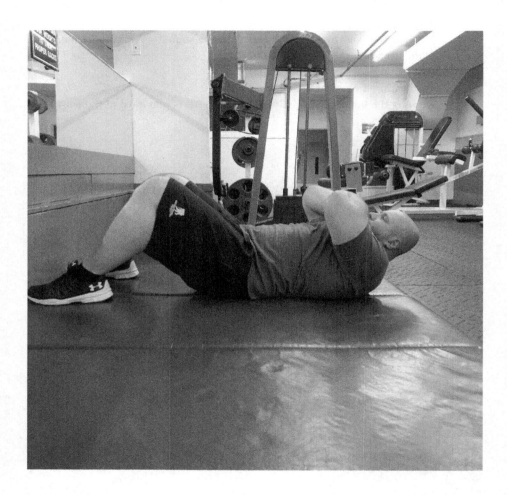

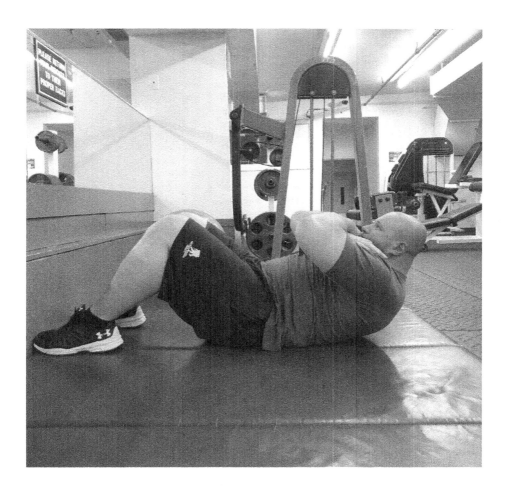

Leg curl

Primary movers: hamstrings.

Secondary movers: calves.

Starting position:

- Lie down on the leg curl machine bench.
- Place your ankles behind the roller pads.
- Grasp the handles to prevent yourself from sliding up and down the bench during the movement.

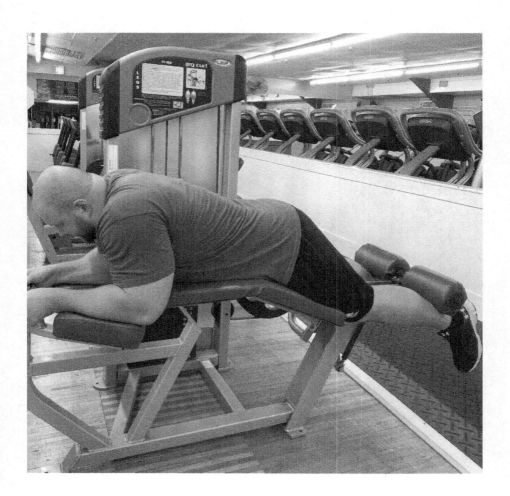

Movement:
- Bend your legs until full knee flexion is achieved.
- Extend your legs back to the starting position under control.
- Stop the descent slightly short of full knee extension.

Common mistakes:
- Not going through full ROM (usually means that the weight is too heavy).
- Allowing your hips to come off of the bench during the exercise.

Caution:
- Avoid the machines that place knees in hyperextension at the starting position.

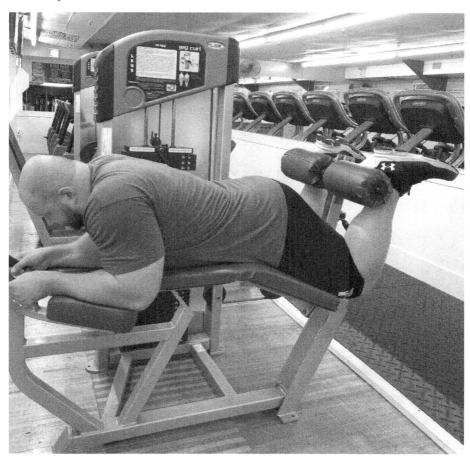

Leg extension

Primary movers: quadriceps.

Starting position:

- Sit in the machine with your back flat against the seat pad.
- Place your ankles behind the roller pads.

Movement:

- Straighten your legs out.
- Lower the weight to the starting position under control.

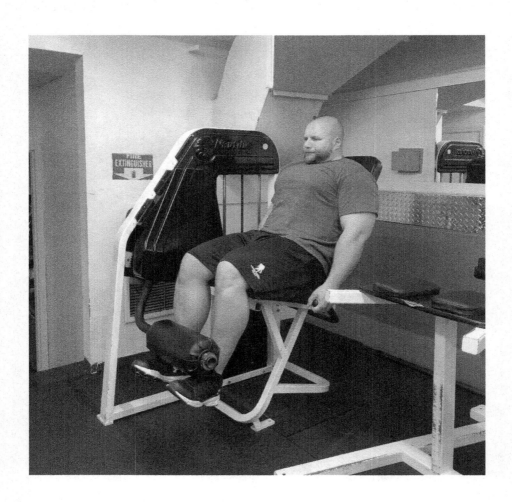

Common mistakes:
- Not going through full ROM.
- Allowing your buttocks to come off of the seat.

Caution:
- Avoid the machines that create very sharp knee angle at the starting position.

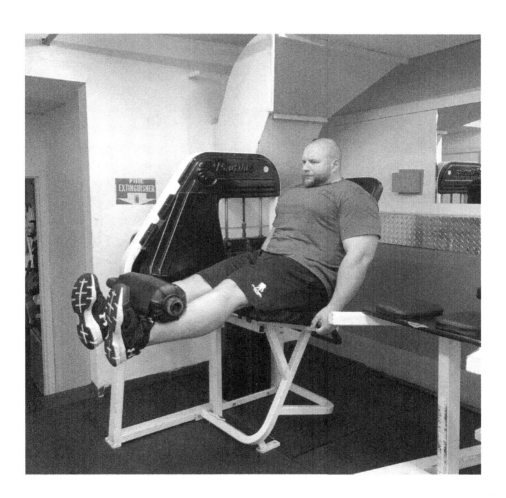

Leg press

Primary movers: quadriceps, gluteus.

Secondary movers: hamstrings, adductors.

Starting position:

- Position yourself in the seat with your back flat against the pad.
- Place your feet on the platform about shoulder width apart with your toes pointing slightly out.
- Unrack the weight on the straight legs and remove the supports.

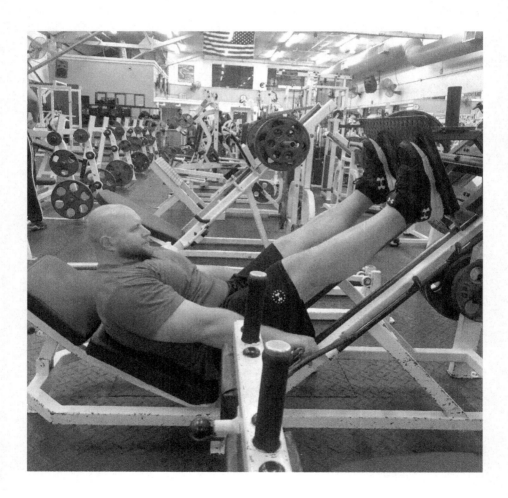

Movement:

- Lower the platform down until your thighs are near the sides of your torso.
- Do not allow your lower back to come off of the seat pad at the bottom position.
- Press the platform back up until your legs are straight, but not hyperextended.
- Make sure that your knees point in the same direction as your feet during both descent and ascent.
- Make sure to maintain even pressure throughout the soles of your feet.

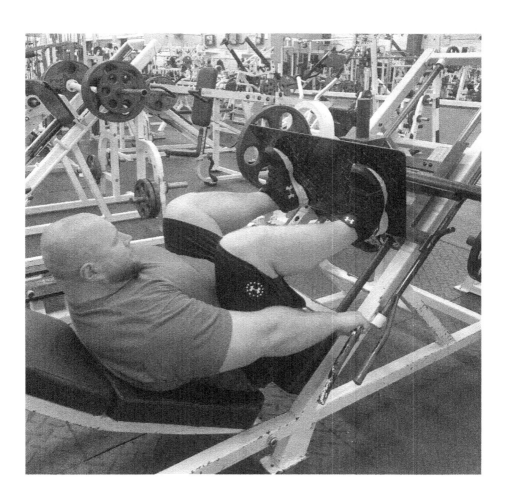

Common mistakes:
- Not going through the full ROM.
- Allowing your lower back to come off of the seat pad (most commonly happens if the feet are positioned too high on the platform).
- Allowing the knees to move inwards on ascent/descent.
- Allowing the heels to come off of the platform at the bottom portion of the movement.

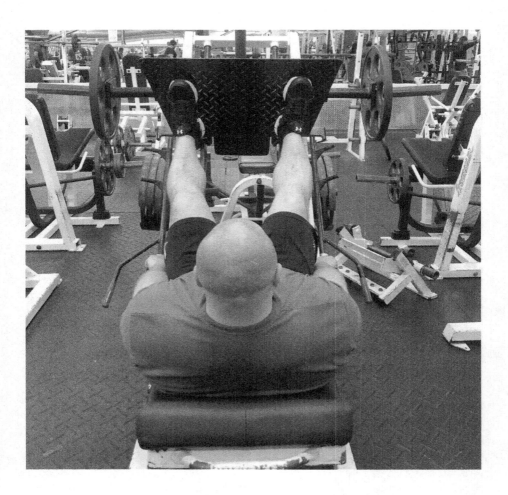

Caution:

- Vertical version of leg press makes it very difficult to keep lower back against the seat at the bottom of the movement and should be considered a poor substitute.

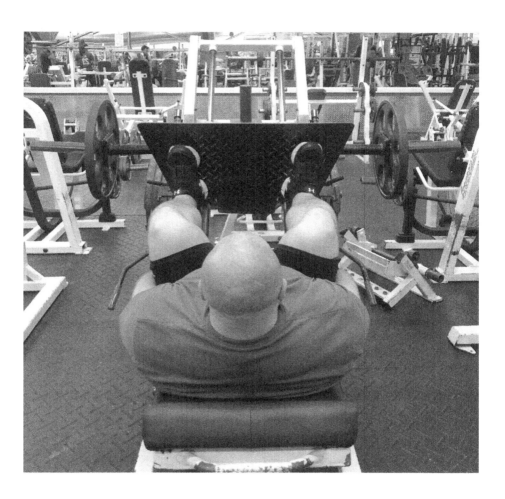

Lunge

Primary movers: quadriceps, gluteus, hamstrings.
Secondary movers: adductors, calves.

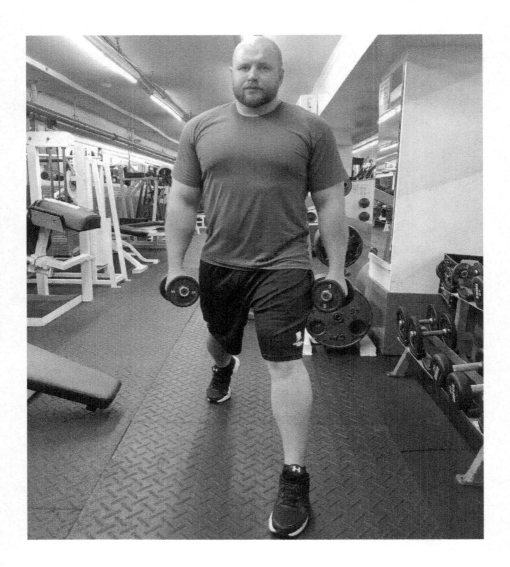

Starting position:
- Position the dumbbells on the side with palms facing each other (if only bodyweight is used, simply place your hands on your hips).
- Make a wide step forward (find a step length at which front leg is just a little past the vertical line at the bottom of the lunge).
- Turn your forward foot slightly inward.

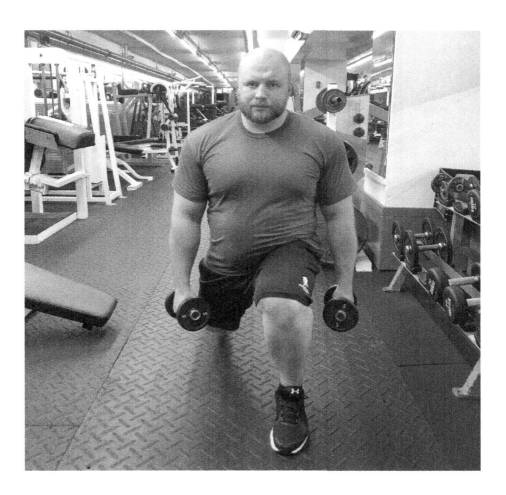

Movement:

- Lower yourself down until the back knee almost touches the floor.
- Bring yourself back up.
- Maintain your torso almost vertical on descent/ascent.
- Make sure your forward knee is aligned with the foot on the descent/ascent.
- Complete all reps on one side before switching to the other leg.

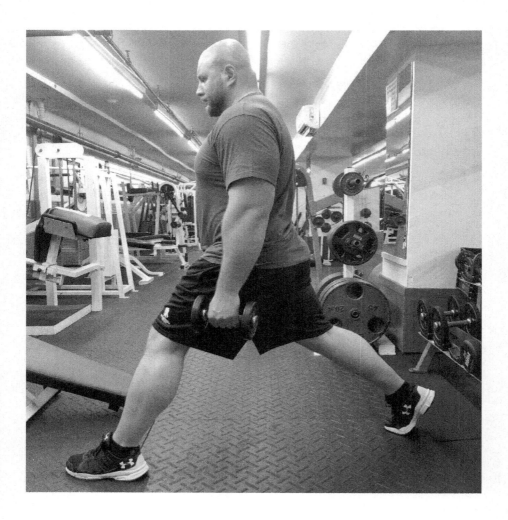

Common mistakes:
- Positioning forward foot straight forward.
- Not lowering down enough (might be due to lack of flexibility).
- Allowing the forward knee to go past the toes at the bottom position.

Alternative:
- It is possible to perform this exercise in alternating fashion (while walking forward) but it requires the reset of the starting position on every rep.

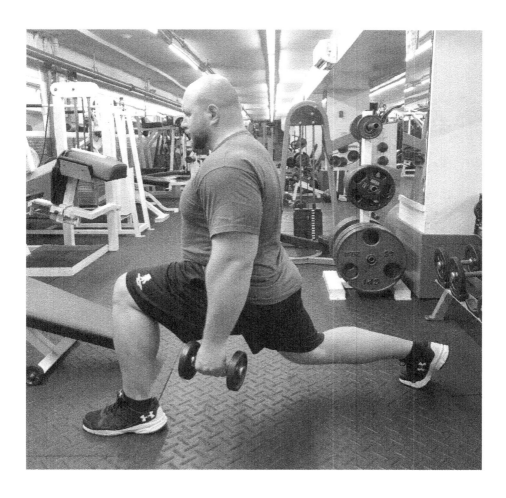

Lying EZ-bar triceps extension

Primary movers: triceps.

Starting position:

- Grasp the bar shoulder width or slightly narrower.
- Lie down on the floor (preferably a mat) or a flat bench.
- Position the bar over your face on straight arms (help of a spotter might be needed to get into starting position).

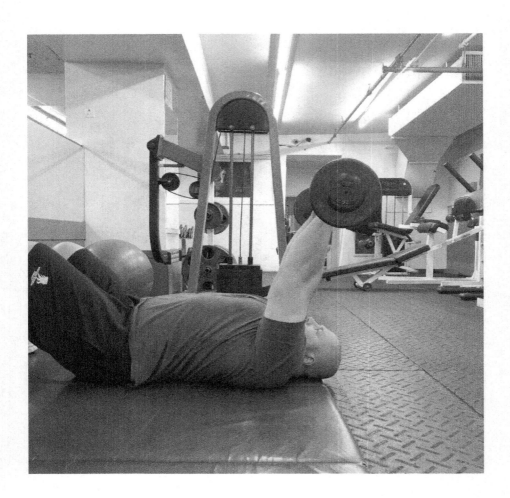

Movement:
- Without any significant movement at the shoulder joints, lower the bar towards your face.
- When the bar gets close to your face, reverse the motion and return back to starting position.
- Ideally only forearms should be moving during this exercise.

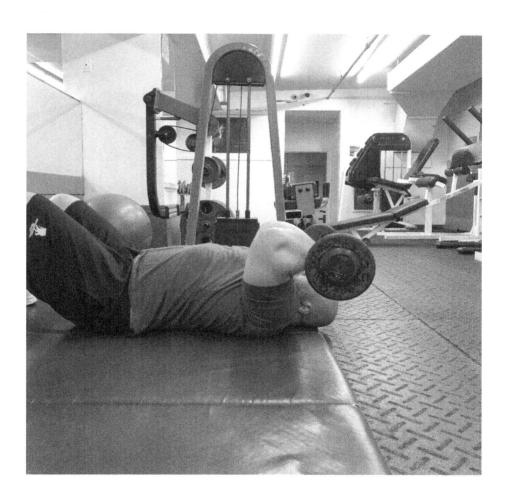

Common mistakes:
- Not going through full ROM.
- Allowing the elbows to flare out to side (which turns exercise into close grip bench press).
- Creating momentum from the bottom position by explosive shoulder extension (as in "Pullover" exercise).

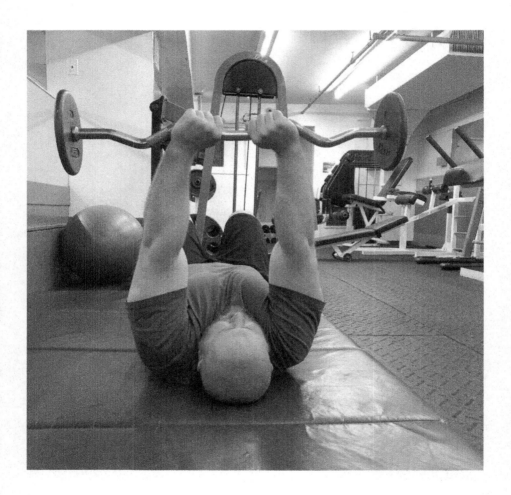

Caution:
- Presence of a spotter is a must when substantial load is being used.

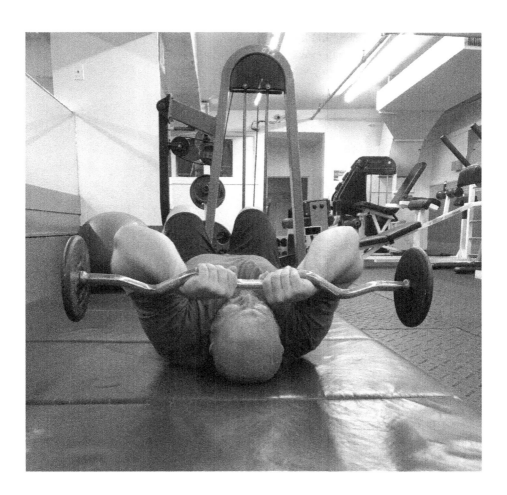

Overhead EZ-bar triceps extension

Primary movers: triceps.

Starting position:

- Stand upright with your feet shoulder width apart.
- Unlock your knees and tighten your lower back in slightly arched position.
- Grasp the bar shoulder width or slightly narrower.
- Position the bar over your head on straight arms.

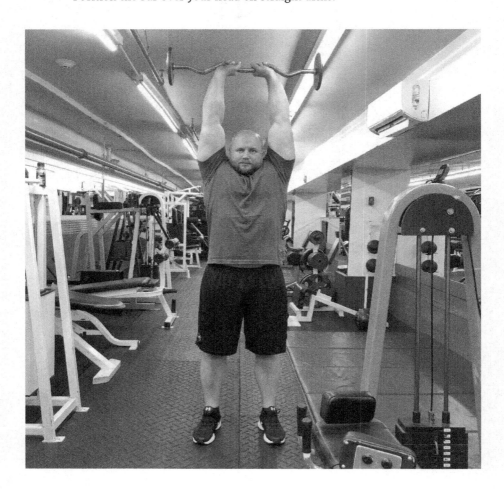

Movement:

- Without too much moment at the shoulder joints, lower the bar behind your head.
- When sufficient triceps stretch is attained, reverse the motion and return back to starting position.
- Ideally only forearms should be moving during this exercise.

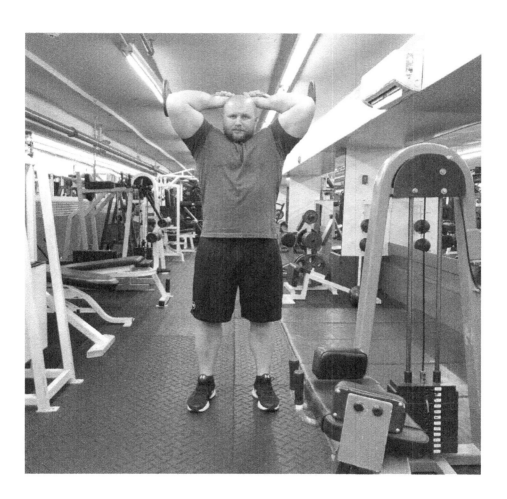

Common mistakes:
- Not going through full ROM.
- Allowing the elbows to flare out to side (which turns exercise into "Behind-The-Neck Press").
- Creating momentum from your legs.

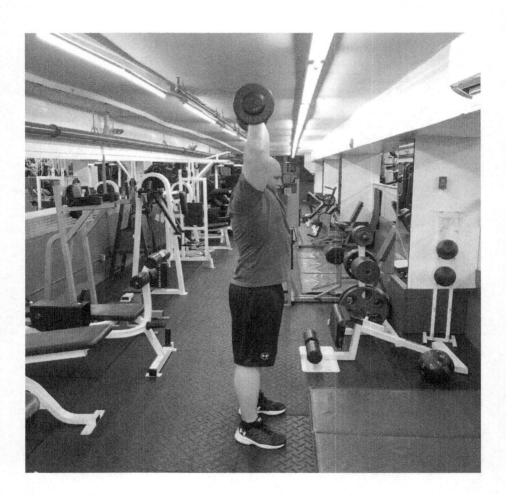

Alternative:

- This exercise can be performed with a dumbbell held in two hands clasped together.

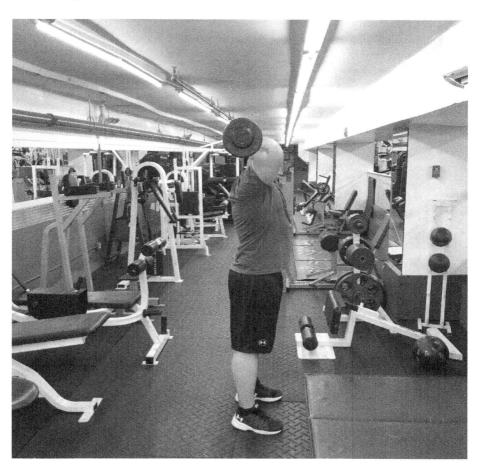

Pull-up

Primary movers: lats.

Secondary movers: biceps, posterior deltoids.

Starting position:

- Position your hands on the bar with shoulder width or wider grip, palms facing forward.
- Hang off of the bar on straight arms and allow your shoulder blades to come slightly out and up.

Movement:

- Pull yourself up while bringing your chest up.

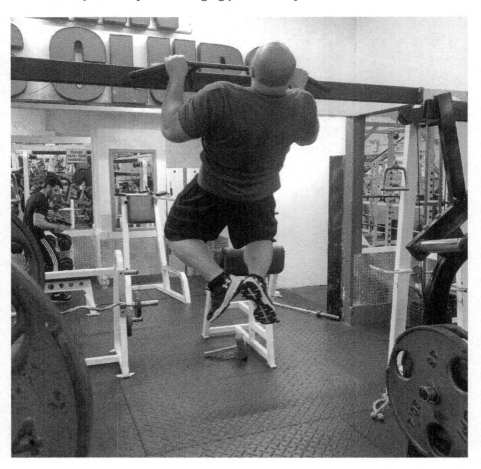

- Try to touch the bar with your chest while squeezing your shoulder blades together.
- Lower yourself under control back to starting position.

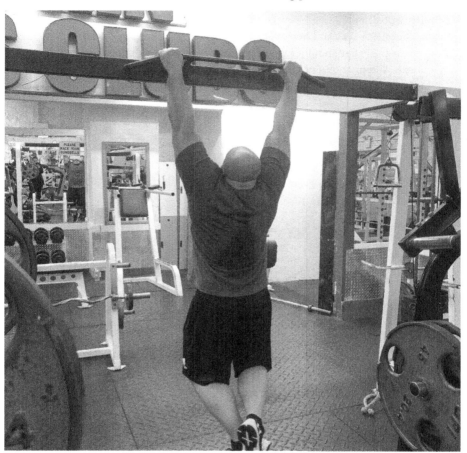

Common mistakes:
- Not going through full ROM.
- Creating momentum by swinging your legs.

Alternative:
- Very wide grip will increase the emphasis on the back musculature (by taking some work away from biceps) but will also decrease the ROM.
- "Kipping Pull-Ups" should not be considered as an alternative for this exercise.

Pulldown

Primary movers: lats.

Secondary movers: biceps, posterior deltoids.

Starting position:

- Sit on the seat and hook your thighs under the roller pads.
- Grasp the bar shoulder width or wider with your palms facing forward.
- Allow your shoulder blades to come slightly out and up
- Your arms should be straight with the bar directly over your head.

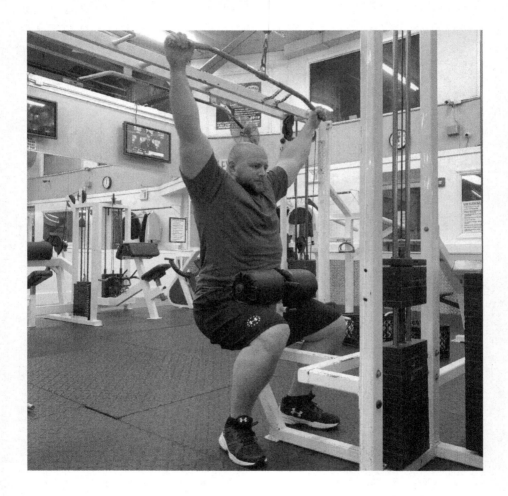

Movement:
- Pull the bar down to your chest while simultaneously raising your chest up.
- Lean back a little during the descent to allow the bar to go past your face.
- Touch your chest with the bar while simultaneously squeezing your shoulder blades together.
- Return the bar back onto outstretched arms.

Common mistakes:
- Not going through full ROM (usually means that the weight is too heavy).
- Creating momentum with explosive back extension.
- Not allowing shoulder blades to come out at the top.
- Not squeezing your shoulder blades together at the bottom.

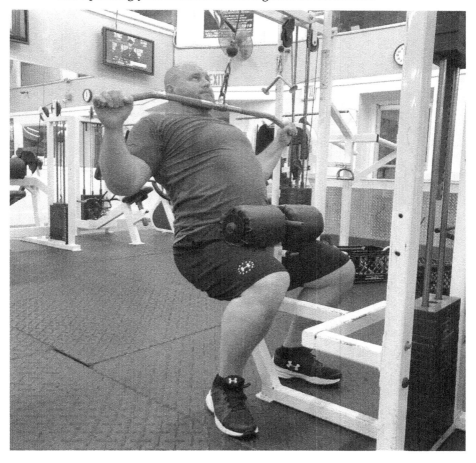

Seated cable row

Primary movers: lats.

Secondary movers: spinal erectors, biceps, posterior deltoids, traps.

Starting position:

- Sit in the seat with your feet positioned on the platform in front of you.
- Tighten your lower back in slightly arched position.
- Bend your knees slightly and maintain that position the whole time.
- Hold the parallel handles with palms facing each other.
- Keep your arms straight and allow your shoulder blades to move slightly out.

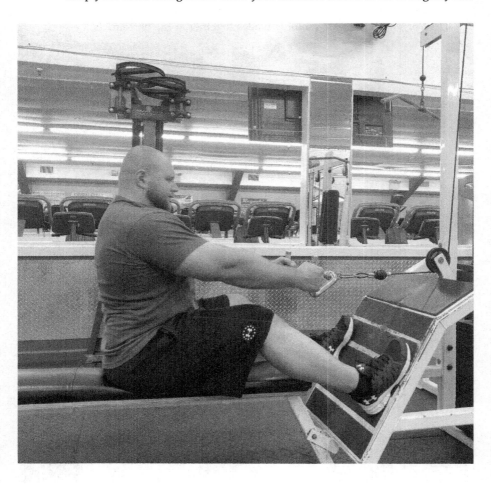

Movement:

- Pull the handles into your belly while sliding your elbows against your ribs.
- Keep your chest up and squeeze your shoulder blades together at the end of the pull.
- Return the weight to the starting position.
- It is natural if your torso moves slightly forward at the beginning of the pull and slightly back at the end of it.

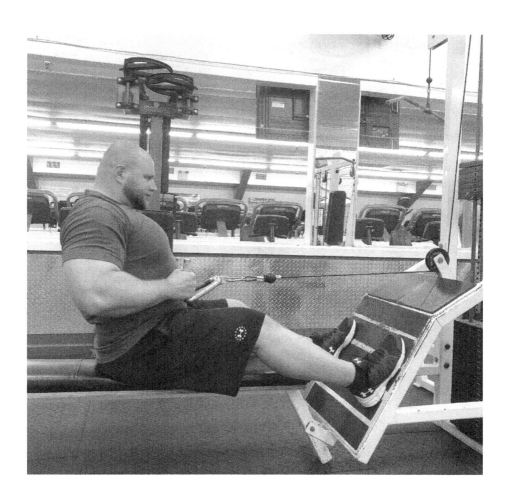

Common mistakes:
- Pulling of the weight towards the chest instead of abdomen.
- Not going through full ROM (usually means that the weight is too heavy).
- Creating momentum with explosive back extension.
- Not allowing shoulder blades to come out in the beginning of the pull.
- Not squeezing your shoulder blades together at the end of the pull.
- Rounding your lower back.

Caution:
- Do not round your lower back when you initially unrack the weight and when you put it back down at the end of a set.

Standing barbell military press

Primary movers: anterior and lateral deltoids.
Secondary movers: triceps, traps.
Starting position:
- Grasp the bar slightly wider than the shoulder width (probably slightly narrower than in bench press) palms facing forward.
- Position the bar in your hands between head line and life line of your palm with thumbs wrapped around.
- Unrack the bar and take two steps back.
- Place your feet about shoulder width apart.
- Keep the bar by your chest (if that creates shoulder discomfort, keep it at about chin level).
- Keep your elbows under the bar.
- Keep your chest high.

Movement:
- Press the bar up and over your head until your arms are straight.
- As soon as the bar is past your face, the head will have to come forward a little.
- Return the bar into starting position.

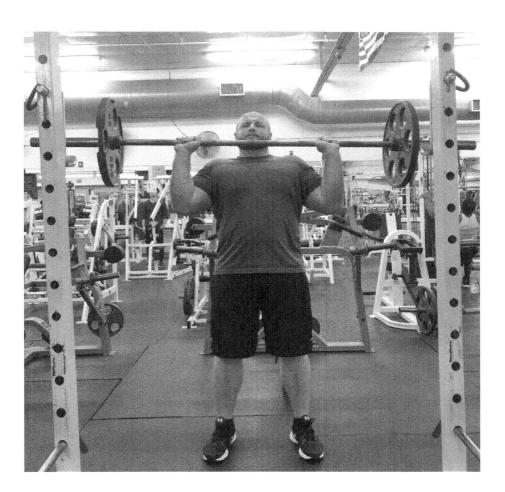

Common mistakes:

- Uneven descent/ascent of the bar.
- Not going through the full ROM.
- Pressing the bar forward instead of over your head.
- Excessive leaning back at the waist during the press.
- Creating momentum with your legs (as in "Push Press" exercise).
- Not maintaining elbows directly under the bar.
- Excessive wrist extension during movement.
- Using thumbless grip.

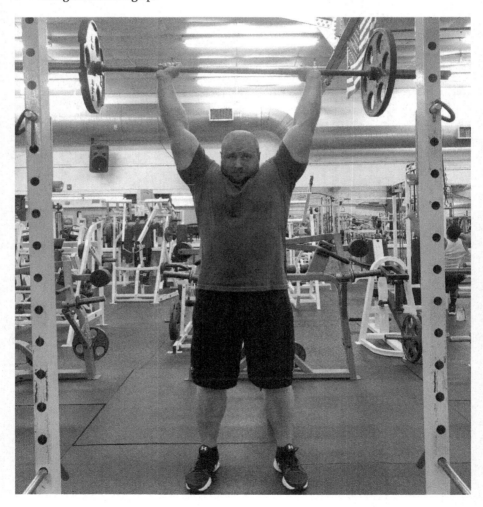

Caution:
- Weightlifting belt could be used for additional back support when very heavy loads are attempted.

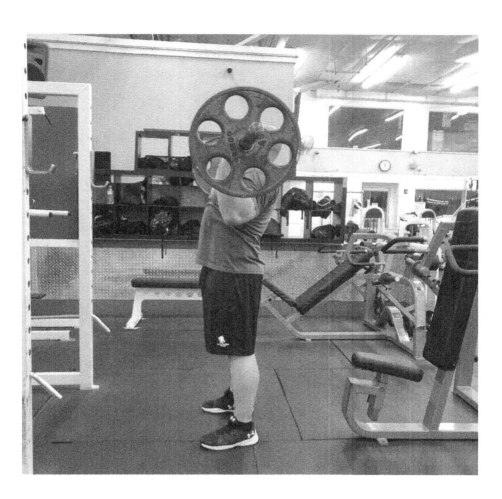

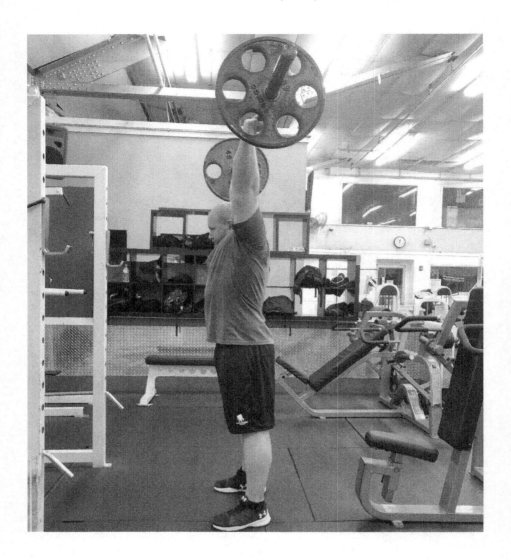

Standing calf raise

Primary movers: calves.

Starting position:

- Stand inside the calf machine with the pads on your shoulders.
- Position the balls of your feet on the step inside the calf machine.
- Unrack the weight and attain an upright position.

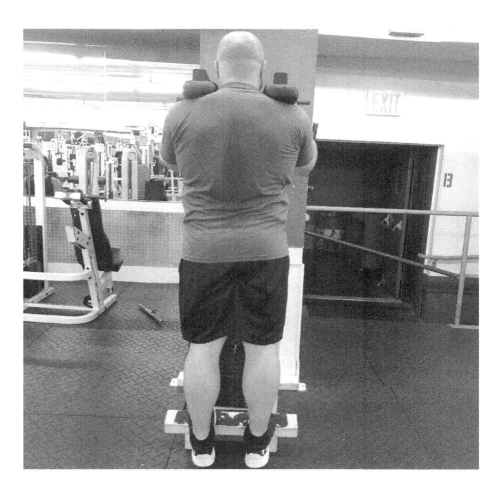

Movement:

- While keeping the knees straight (but not hyperextended), lower your heels down until good gastrocnemius stretch is attained.
- Bring yourself up on your toes as high as possible.

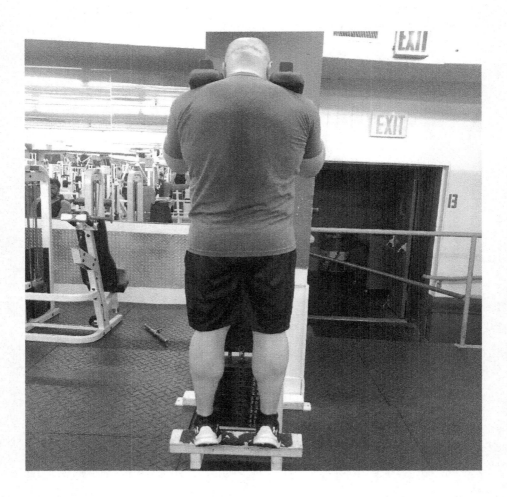

Common mistakes:
- Not going through full ROM (usually means that the weight is too heavy).
- Performing short squats instead of plantarflexion/dorsiflexion.

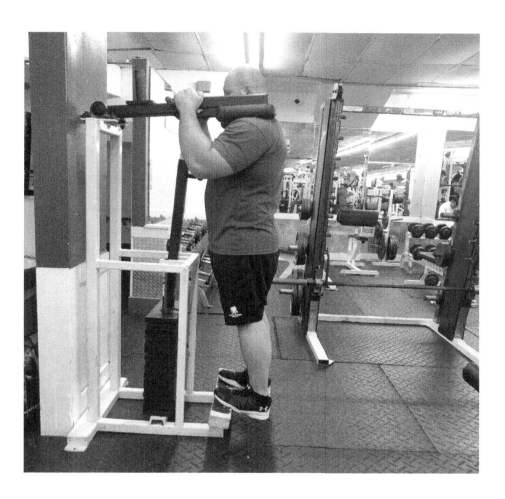

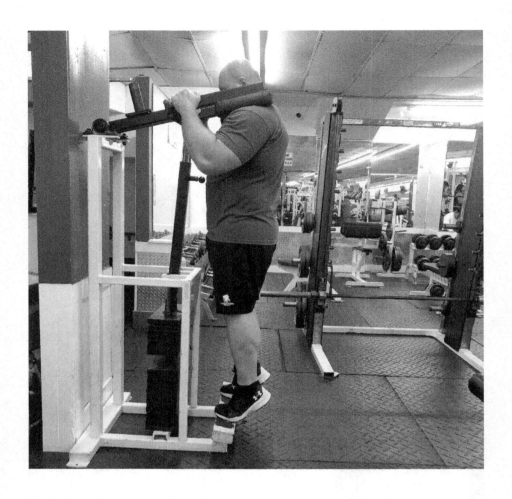

Standing dumbbell lateral raise

Primary movers: lateral and anterior deltoids.

Secondary movers: traps.

Starting position:

- Stand upright with your feet about shoulder width apart.
- Unlock your knees and tighten your lower back in slightly arched position.
- Position dumbbells in front of your upper thighs with palms facing each other.
- Maintain slight bent at your elbows.

Movement:

- Raise dumbbells to the side stopping at about eye level.

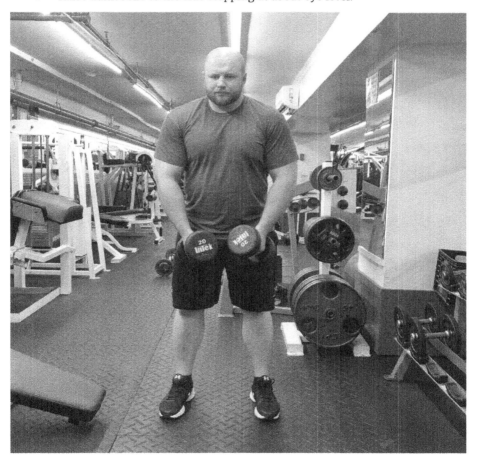

- Lower dumbbells to the starting position under control.
- The only place significant movement should occur during this exercise is the shoulder joint.

Common mistakes:
- Elbows are excessively bent.
- Not going through full ROM (usually because the weight is too heavy).
- Swinging the weight up with momentum created from legs and back.

Caution:
- Turning your thumbs down (pointing to the floor) at the top position puts a lot of additional stress on shoulder joints.

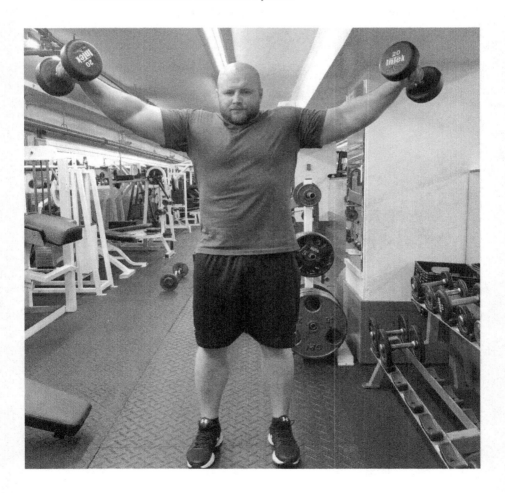

Patience

Always strive for perfection when it comes to exercise execution. Sloppy form might allow you to increase the loads faster initially, but will unavoidably hinder your progress in a long run. Let me illustrate. We will use example with the barbell curls.

Let's say it's your first time doing this exercise. Your buddies are at the gym and it would be pretty embarrassing to start with an empty bar. 25 pound plate on each side makes it look a lot better. It is clearly too heavy but you "ain't no quitter." You raise your elbows and lean backwards a little. Didn't get all the reps required but "at least you tried." Your biceps are fine next day. Just the elbows are a little sore.

You remember about progressive overload at the next session. But who uses small plates? Let's add 10s on each side (115 total). Initially you can't move it even one inch. But then you figure out that if you swing it with your torso hard enough, you might just be able to catch it at the top. Your biceps are almost completely uninvolved at this point, but you are all about "embracing the grind." The elbows are really hurting by the end of the session. But it's okay. It is time for the elbow sleeves anyway. Just don't forget to get a matching baseball cap. It makes you look kind of serious.

You thinking about adding just 5 pounds on each side this time, but here is the thing – it is time to post something on Snapchat. 45 it is! You just have to save some energy by skipping the warm up. You are already used to the elbow pain, but now the lower back also feels kind of weird. No problem. That's what weightlifting belts are for, right?

You are "paying your dues" for the next few weeks but your biceps are not growing. Instead, aches all over your body becoming a bit of a problem. Angry and frustrated you tell your friends "This stupid program doesn't work! Time to get some "roids" yo!"

The above example might seem kind of comical. But those who stuck around at the gym long enough will tell you that it's not that far from reality. 99% of people at 99% of gyms have no idea what they are doing.

People are not patient enough to learn the proper exercise technique. They are not disciplined enough to stay with small consistent weight increases. Some will even be too lazy to read this little book all the way to the end. The result: thousands (maybe millions) of gym members that don't look like they have ever trained at all. Not to mention all the injuries guys manage to get while still training at the beginner's level of performance.

PROGRAMMING

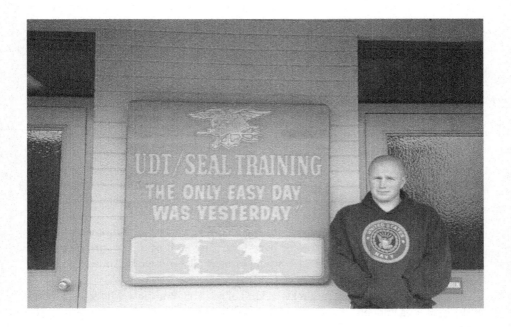

"Success occurs when opportunity meets preparation."
– Zig Ziglar

If you decided to get right down to business and skipped to this part – go back. Without understanding of some basic methodology these programs might not appear much different from anything you can put together yourself. It is not just "I pick things up and put them down" here. Every little detail is there for a reason and you should know what that reason is.

Expression "the whole is greater than the sum of its parts" definitely applies to training programs. You can't just take random parts from different cars, throw them in a pile and call it an automobile. Similarly, mindless bunching of different exercises together does not mean you created a training program.

That is not to say that the information presented here is magical. This book is simply a map that shows you the shortest way to being big and strong. But you still have to make this journey (i.e. do all the hard work) by yourself.

Overall structure

"Big and Strong" training system is based on rotation of strength and hypertrophy phases. This method of structuring the training process is called *block periodization*. Both phases are designed to complement each other. As you get stronger in the strength phase (SP) you should be able to lift slightly heavier weights in the following hypertrophy phase (HP). This should lead to muscle growth. Which in turn should help you to increase the weights once you get back to the SP. So on and so forth. You will spend 3 to 6 weeks (usually 4) in each phase while alternating them continuously.

As you already know, the main purpose of periodization is to maintain variability of training. But don't discount the importance of staying mentally fresh. Monotony will cut down even the most enthusiastic trainees. It is also a lot easier to do your best when you see the light at the end of the tunnel. Just think about running a race: you push especially hard when you know that the finish line is near.

During the first week of each phase you will purposely significantly lower the intensity. The reason for that is to allow your body to fully recover from the most intense last few weeks of the previous phase. As we discussed in our "energy budget" theory, going to battle every time you are in the gym is very courageous but, unfortunately, cannot be sustained for too long. Planned periods of relatively easy workouts are referred to as **deload**s and are commonly used in strength training.

Another reason to reduce the load in the beginning of each phase is to gain some momentum before hitting your previous best. Different phases do not contain all the same exercises and they are performed in different modes. Therefore, some time is need to transition an increase in one athletic quality into another (remember transformation).

Your short term goal is to always finish each phase with at least some improvements in your performance in all (or at least some) exercises. Strive to either complete more reps (while staying within prescribed ranges) with the same weight or to use heavier weight while keeping reps constant.

Be mindful that you won't be comparing consecutive phases. Loads and reps you were able to complete on the last week of strength phase will be compared to the ones you achieved in the same exercises on the last week of the previous strength phase. Loads and reps you were able to complete on the last week of hypertrophy phase will be compared to the ones you achieved in the same exercises on the last week of the previous hypertrophy phase.

Due to accommodation, the amount of progress during each phase will ultimately depend on the level of your qualification. The beginners might need only a few light initial sessions and be ready to move forward for the rest of the phase. The more advanced, on the other hand, might need to take three weeks just to get to their previous best and then try to beat it only on the last week.

Every three to six months you can take a week off from training. Obviously, it is better to schedule these breaks during occasions such as family vacation. Also, make sure you earn your breaks by training especially hard in the preceding weeks (concept often referred to as **overreaching**). Here is an example of how training process could be structured:

SP (4 weeks) → HP (4 weeks) → SP (4 weeks) → HP (5 weeks) → week off → SP (4 weeks) → HP (4 weeks) → SP (3 weeks) → ...

Strength phase

This phase is all about getting stronger and the focus is on mechanical tension. SP contains nothing but the best compound free weight movements. Every training session is a whole body workout. Rest breaks between sets should be around 2-3 minutes. The speed of the exercises is explosive but the proper form must be maintained.

Odd Weeks

MONDAY – 1A	WEDNESDAY – 1B	FRIDAY – 1C
Barbell bench press 5x5	Deadlift 5x5	Barbell bench press 5x5
Back squat 5x5	Barbell bench press 5x5	Back squat 5x5
Standing barbell military press 5x5	Barbell bent-over row 5x5	Standing barbell military press 5x5

Even weeks

MONDAY – 2A	WEDNESDAY – 2B	FRIDAY – 2C
Back squat 5x5	Barbell bench press 5x5	Back squat 5x5
Barbell bench press 5x5	Deadlift 5x5	Barbell bench press 5x5
Barbell bent-over row 5x5	Standing barbell military press 5x5	Barbell bent-over row 5x5

It is perfectly fine if you are unable to train on the days of the week specified above. When you create a schedule that works best for you, make sure there is a day off in between every training session (Friday-A/Sunday-B/Tuesday-C). Also, training session C and A should have two days in between them.

Hypertrophy phase

This phase is a bodybuilding style training and it's all about metabolic stress. HP contains both compound and isolation exercises that are arranged by muscle groups (*split routine*). The rest breaks between sets should be around 60 -90 seconds. The speed of exercises is slower with mental focus on muscle contraction.

MONDAY - A	TUESDAY – B	THURSDAY – C	SATURDAY – D
Barbell bench press 3x12-8	Leg extension 3x12-8	Standing dumbbell lateral raise 3x12-8	Pull-up 3x12-8
Incline dumbbell press 3x12-8	Leg press 3x12-8	Standing barbell military press 3x12-8	Barbell bent-over row 3x12-8
Dip 3x12-8	Back squat 3x12-8	Overhead EZ-bar triceps extension 3x12-8	Deadlift 3x12-8
Barbell biceps curl 3x12-8	Leg curl 3x12-8	Close grip barbell bench press 3x12-8	Dumbbell shrug 3x12-8
Dumbbell hammer curl 3x12-8	Standing calf raise 3X12-8	Incline sit-up 3x20-15	Bent-over dumbbell raise 3x12-8

If you can't train on the days listed above, feel free to make adjustments. Do your best, however, to spread training sessions as much as possible throughout the week. Ideally only A and B sessions should fall on consecutive days (Saturday-A/Sunday-B/Tuesday-C/Thursday-D). Also, make sure not to schedule workout A on the very next day after workout D.

Progression

Increasing the MTLs used is the key progression of this training system. It should not, however, be done at the expense of proper form of exercise execution. The reps that were performed with improper technique or required assistance from your training partner are not to be counted. Also, keep in mind that the discussion below does not include the warm-up sets.

We are going to use squat to illustrate the progression. During SP squat is performed twice a week (Monday and Friday in our example). Let's say on Monday of week 1 you used 135lbs and were able to perform 5 sets of 5 reps. This means that for the following Friday you can increase the MTL for squat by 5 or 10 pounds. Let's say you went up to 145 and were able to get 5x5 again. Then for the following squat session you can increase the weight by 5 to 10 pounds, once again.

On Monday of the second week you used 155, but this time were able to get only 5, 5, 5, 4, 4. This means that you should stay with that MTL for another training session (Friday of the second week). Let's say that Friday you were able to complete 5 reps in all five sets. It is time to increase MTL again. On Monday of week three you went for 165 and got 5, 5, 4, 4, 3 reps. As you might have already guessed, we will be staying with 165 for the following Friday.

Let's say on that Friday you improve to 5, 5, 5, 5, 4, 4 and on the Monday of week four you finally get 5x5. Now you are clear to go up in weight again, use your discretion though. Since things are toughening up, maybe it is reasonable to increase weight only by 5 pounds now. This way for the Friday of week four perhaps you should only go up to 170.

Even with such a small increase that session was probably a battle. Good news – the strength phase is over. When we switch to HP, it is only logical that MTLs have to be reduced due to higher reps and shorter rest breaks. In HP the focus is primarily on getting maximum pump, which makes it a perfect time to give your mind and your joints a break from heavy weights.

We are going to continue using squat for further illustration. During hypertrophy phases every exercise is performed only once a week. Let's say you decided to use 115 for you first HP squat work out and completed 12, 11 and 10 reps.

This is still good enough to try to increase the MTL next time. As long as you get at least ten reps or above in all sets.

Let's say you used 125 on the second week and did 12, 10, and 8. Based on that performance it would be reasonable to stay with that weight for week three. If this time you were able to complete 12, 12 and 10, for week four you could attempt 135. As the burn in your quads is getting worse with every session, you might just be missing SP by now.

When you get back to SP, allow yourself to "deload" and then gain some momentum before hitting your previous best. 135 for 5x5 for the first session should feel pretty easy. For the second session use 155 to make transition smother before hitting the 170 on the week two.

Hopefully the above illustration made it clear how beneficial the training log is. It is very difficult to remember all reps and sets for every exercise. Accurate training log will allow you to see how you are progressing from session to session and from one phase to another. "Big and Strong" app is specifically designed to help you keep records for training programs presented here.

Total beginners

Trainees with zero resistance training experience will need to reduce the overall volume initially and then slowly increase it as their work capacity improves. Don't jump ahead of yourself just to prove that you are a special case.

Regardless of your genetic predisposition, nobody is going to look like Arnold Schwarzenegger after just a few months of training. Imagine that you used Formula 1 car to learn how to drive. Chances are you would probably get seriously hurt. Similarly, nothing good is going to happen if you skip right to the more advanced programs presented here.

When you just start training your main goal is to learn proper technique of exercises. To make this process easier it is best to focus only on the few main moves, which makes SP perfect for beginners. If you don't have anyone experienced supervising you, periodically videotape yourself from different angles to analyze your technique.

Pay attention to developing rhythmical breathing patterns while learning new exercises. Compound movements that require stabilization of torso might require brief holding of breath while getting through "sticking" points, especially when heavy loads are used. However, care must be taken to make sure that this is not done excessively, as such practices put a lot of strain on cardiovascular system.

Also remember that no exercise should be causing an excruciating pain. Because if it does – stop and assess the situation. Either you are performing it incorrectly or there is an underlying pathology that needs to be checked out by a qualified healthcare professional. In either case take appropriate measures right away.

As you learn each new exercise, start with an empty bar and perform five reps while focusing on proper execution of the lift. If everything goes well, add 10-20 pounds and do another set. You can repeat the process for the total of 3 to 5 sets:

1st set: 45lbs 5 reps (warm-up)
2nd set: 55lbs 5 reps (warm-up)
3rd set: 65lbs 3 reps (work)

It is important to stay PATIENT with these weight increases. We are not trying to set a new world record here. The priority is learning the proper form. *Faulty patterns learned in the initial stages of training are very difficult to correct later on.* Another reason to be prudent during the first few training sessions is to avoid unnecessarily severe muscle soreness during the following days.

Once you reach the weight with which you were not able to complete 5 reps with correct technique, you will move on to the next exercise of the session. Therefore, the heaviest set in each exercise will be the only work set you will perform. With each successive training session you will try to work your way up to a slightly heavier weight in each exercise:

1st set: 45lbs 5 reps
2nd set: 55lbs 5 reps
3rd set: 65lbs 5 reps
4th set: 75lbs 4 reps

You will stick to this model for the duration of Strength Phase as you go through it for the first time. Similar approach will be taken when you start your first Hypertrophy Phase in few weeks. The number of different exercises will be higher, but at that point you already have some idea of what you are doing at the gym. Also, instead of working your way up in weight in sets of five, you will be using sets of 12 here.

If you are not able to perform the required number of pull-ups, temporarily substitute them with pulldowns. Similarly, employ assisted dip machine until you are able to perform dips on your own. Ultimately you should be able to perform both of these exercises with additional weight.

When you go through SP for the second time, start performing two sets of five reps with the heaviest weight for that session in each exercise:

1st set: 45lbs 5 reps
2nd set: 95lbs 5 reps
3rd set: 135lbs 5 reps
4th set: 185lbs 5 reps
5th set: 185lbs 5 reps

If you were able to get five reps in both sets, increase the weight by 5-10 pounds at the next session. At this point you will start switching to the overload method described in "Progression" chapter. With each subsequent Strength Phase you will add one work set until you reach five (not counting warm-ups). The same thing goes for Hypertrophy Phases, only here you will stop adding when you reach three work sets:

1st month (SP): warm-up + 1 set of 5 reps
2nd month (HP): warm-up + 1 set of 12 reps
3rd month (SP): warm-up + 2 sets of 5 reps
4th month (HP): warm-up + 2 sets of 12 reps
5th month (SP): warm-up + 3 sets of 5 reps
6th month (HP): warm-up + 3 sets of 12 reps
7th month (SP): warm-up + 4 sets of 5 reps
8th month (HP): warm-up + 3 sets of 12 reps
9th month (SP): warm-up + 5 sets of 5 reps
10th month (HP): warm-up + 3 sets of 12 reps

You can stay with 5 sets of 5 reps in Strength Phases for as long as you are able to slowly increase the weight on the bar. You will quickly realize that it is a lot easier in squats and deadlifts. In these two exercises you will probably be able to increase MTLs by 10 pounds at a time, at least initially. For the rest, 5 pound jumps might be more appropriate.

Once increasing of the weight becomes obviously stagnant, you can switch to the model of decreasing reps from week to week (5X6, 5X5, 5X4, 5X3), as shown below. This is a slightly more complex way to organize training process as it requires some experience to estimate appropriate weight for the reps prescribed for each week.

Week 1

MONDAY – 1A	WEDNESDAY – 1B	FRIDAY – 1C
Barbell bench press 5x6	Deadlift 5x6	Barbell bench press 5x6
Back squat 5x6	Barbell bench press 5x6	Back squat 5x6
Standing barbell military press 5x6	Barbell bent-over row 5x6	Standing barbell military press 5x6

Week 2

MONDAY – 2A	WEDNESDAY – 2B	FRIDAY – 2C
Back squat 5x5	Barbell bench press 5x5	Back squat 5x5
Barbell bench press 5x5	Deadlift 5x5	Barbell bench press 5x5
Barbell bent-over row 5x5	Standing barbell military press 5x5	Barbell bent-over row 5x5

Week 3

MONDAY – 1A	WEDNESDAY – 1B	FRIDAY – 1C
Barbell bench press 5x4	Deadlift 5x4	Barbell bench press 5x4
Back squat 5x4	Barbell bench press 5x4	Back squat 5x4
Standing barbell military press 5x4	Barbell bent-over row 5x4	Standing barbell military press 5x4

Week 4

MONDAY – 2A	WEDNESDAY – 2B	FRIDAY – 2C
Back squat 5x3	Barbell bench press 5x3	Back squat 5x3
Barbell bench press 5x3	Deadlift 5x3	Barbell bench press 5x3
Barbell bent-over row 5x3	Standing barbell military press 5x3	Barbell bent-over row 5x3

Intermediate level

Intermediate category includes trainees with more than a year of well-structured training. At this point further modifications might be necessary to ensure continuing progress. One of the ways to do it during Strength Phases is by employing rotation of high volume and high intensity days, similar to the *Texas Method*. Volume day will be considered a training session when you perform your usual five work sets in an exercise (for the number of reps assigned for that week). On the intensity day you will work up to the repetition maximum (RM) for the number of reps assigned for that week and will complete only one set with that weight.

Since on every intensity day (with exception of the first week or so) you will be attempting to set a new personal record (PR) for a particular number of reps, it is better not to overexert yourself on the volume days. Some experimentation will be required to find the level of effort of the volume workout that prepares you optimally for the following intensity workout. Also, keep in mind that volume and intensity sessions will not fall on the same days for different exercises.

For example, for squats Mondays would be intensity days and Fridays would be volume days. For bench press I would recommend to schedule intensity days on the days when this exercise falls in the beginning of the training session. For deadlifts you will only have intensity days and, therefore, will be performing only one work set in this exercise per week. On the contrary, for shoulder presses and barbell rows you will only have volume days and will continue doing five work sets at every training session.

Week 1

MONDAY – 1A	WEDNESDAY – 1B	FRIDAY – 1C
Barbell bench press 1x6RM	Deadlift 1x6RM	Barbell bench press 1x6RM
Back squat 1x6RM	Barbell bench press 5x6	Back squat 5x6
Standing barbell military press 5x6	Barbell bent-over row 5x6	Standing barbell military press 5x6

Week 2

MONDAY – 2A	WEDNESDAY – 2B	FRIDAY – 2C
Back squat 1x5RM	Barbell bench press 1x5RM	Back squat 5x5
Barbell bench press 5x5	Deadlift 1x5RM	Barbell bench press 5x5
Barbell bent-over row 5x5	Standing barbell military press 5x5	Barbell bent-over row 5x5

Week 3

MONDAY – 1A	WEDNESDAY – 1B	FRIDAY – 1C
Barbell bench press 1x4RM	Deadlift 1x4RM	Barbell bench press 1x4RM
Back squat 1x4RM	Barbell bench press 5x4	Back squat 5x4
Standing barbell military press 5x4	Barbell bent-over row 5x4	Standing barbell military press 5x4

Week 4

MONDAY – 2A	WEDNESDAY – 2B	FRIDAY – 2C
Back squat 1x3RM	Barbell bench press 1x3RM	Back squat 5x3
Barbell bench press 5x3	Deadlift 1x3RM	Barbell bench press 5x3
Barbell bent-over row 5x3	Standing barbell military press 5x3	Barbell bent-over row 5x3

When it comes to Hypertrophy phases the modifications could be applied to the whole phase or only to exercises for a particular muscle group. You can experiment with either reps or sets. For example, try sets of 15 reps in all leg exercises in the upcoming HP. Or, if you want to emphasize biceps during one of the hypertrophy phases, increase work sets in exercises for this muscle as the phase progresses:

1st week: 3x12-8

2nd week: 4x12-8

3rd week: 5x12-8

4th week: 6x12-8

Be very careful with anything that requires significant overall volume increase. Even the original version of HP presents a significant challenge to your recovery capabilities and cramming more work into it could push things over the edge. Therefore, while prioritizing a lagging body part, it might be wise to reduce the workload for some of your stronger ones. For example, perform only one work set in all back exercises during the same phase when you are bombarding your biceps.

Strength phase 2

This variation of the strength phase could be used as alternative for SP. All the core principles of the strength phase remain the same. The main difference is that SP2 utilizes broader range of exercises.

MONDAY – A	WEDNESDAY – B	FRIDAY – C
Back squat 5x4	Hang power clean 5x4	Front squat 5x4
Barbell bench press 5x5	Standing barbell military press 5x5	Dip 5x5
Chin-up 5x6	Deadlift 5x6	Barbell bent-over row 5x6

Hypertrophy phase 2

This is another training program that could be used in hypertrophy phase. HP2 combines both strength and hypertrophy modes of training. Such training approach is called *concurrent periodization* method and has become increasingly popular in powerlifting in recent years. Also, you will be resting 2-3 minutes between the sets of the first exercise of each session and 60-90 seconds for the rest. "5/3/1 Forever" by Jim Wendler can give you countless ideas on how similar training templates can be modified in many different ways.

MONDAY – A	TUESDAY – B	THURSDAY – C	SATURDAY – D
Barbell bench press 5x5	Back squat 5x5	Standing barbell military press 5x5	Deadlift 5x5
Seated dumbbell press 3x12-8	Barbell bent-over row 3x12-8	Incline dumbbell press 3x12-8	Leg press 3x12-8
Lying EZ-bar triceps extension 3x12-8	Barbell biceps curl 3x12-8	Close grip barbell bench press 3x12-8	Dumbbell shrug 3x12-8
Dip 3x12-8	Standing calf raise 3x12-8	Incline sit-up 3x20-15	Pull-up 3x12-8

Utilizing the above alternative phases in addition to all other modifications presented in this section will give you enough tools for many years of successful training. More advanced athletes can further increase variability by incorporating new exercises. The best way to do that is by substituting prescribed exercises with similar variations without changing the overall structure of the programs. For example, you could do seated calf raises during one hypertrophy phase and standing during the next. Or you could do conventional deadlift in hypertrophy phases and sumo style during strength phases.

Athletes who are getting closer to the advanced level can start introducing tools such as chains, bands, boards etc. "Book of Methods" by Louie Simmons presents many ways how such modalities can be employed during strength phases. As far as hypertrophy phases, these athletes can start CAREFUL experimentation with the intensification techniques presented in "Reps and Sets" section. Good old "Encyclopedia of Modern Bodybuilding" is a great reference for more of the muscle building tricks.

Advanced training program

If you don't have at least two or three years of training experience, I would suggest that you skip this section for now. Only **advanced** athletes (and perhaps **advanced intermediates**) require this level of programming complexity. Advanced training program (ATP) is based on *undulating periodization* model. Due to built-in variability, it can be utilized slightly longer than your usual four weeks.

When using ATP you will be training three times a week while rotating two exercise complexes (A and B). ATP also employs a three stage microcycle: heavy day, light day and moderate day. Since each complex is performed three times in two weeks, the full microcycle takes two weeks:

Odd Weeks

MONDAY - A	WEDNESDAY - B	FRIDAY - A
Barbell bench press 5x2 (100%)	Deadlift 5x4 (90%)	Barbell bench press 5x6 (80%)
Back squat 5x2 (100%)	Standing barbell military press 5x4 (90%)	Back squat 5x6 (80%)
Dip 5x2 (100%)	Barbell bent-over row 5x4 (90%)	Dip 5x6 (80%)

Even Weeks

MONDAY - B	WEDNESDAY - A	FRIDAY - B
Deadlift 5x2 (100%)	Barbell bench press 5x4 (90%)	Deadlift 5x6 (80%)
Standing barbell military press 5x2 (100%)	Back squat 5x4 (90%)	Standing barbell military press 5x6 (80%)
Barbell bent-over row 5x2 (100%)	Dip 5x4 (90%)	Barbell bent-over row 5x6 (80%)

Let's stick to complex A for illustration. We will assume that your training schedule is Monday, Wednesday and Friday. Every microcycle begins with the "heavy" day (Monday in our example). On "heavy" days you perform 5 sets of 2 reps in all exercises (not counting warm-ups). The MTLs you use in exercises on "heavy" days will be considered to be 100% for the rest of this microcycle. Once again, 100% here does not mean your 1RM.

The next time you perform complex A will be on Friday. Friday's are "light" days. On "light" days you perform 5 sets of 6 reps in all exercises. The MTLs you use here will be 80% of the weights you used on previous Monday. So simply multiply Monday's MTLs for each exercise of complex A by 0.8.

Your third complex A workout will fall on Wednesday of the following week. Wednesdays are "moderate" days. The MTLs you use here will be 90% of the weights you used on the Monday of the week before. So simply multiple those weights by 0.9. You will perform 5 sets of 4 reps with the multiplication products for the respective exercises. This will complete this microcycle for complex A.

Successful completion of all prescribed sets and reps in any of the exercises of the microcycle allows you to increase the MTLs in those exercises for the following "heavy" day. Depending on how comfortable MTL felt for 5x2 in that particular exercise on the previous "heavy" day (two weeks ago), you can add 5-10 pounds to it. Now this new MTL will be considered as 100% for this exercise for the new microcycle. Therefore, the MTLs for "light" and "moderate" day will change accordingly.

All this might sound incredibly complicated but once you get the idea it is actually pretty simple. We will use Back Squat to illustrate. Let's say you want to use 405lbs for you first "heavy" day. This means that after proper warm up you will perform 5 sets of two reps with that MTL. The following Friday is a "light" day and you will use 80% of your "heavy" day MTL:

405 x 0.8 = 324lbs

This means you will squat 5 sets of 6 reps with 324lbs. The next time you do squats is on Wednesday of the following week. Wednesdays are the "moderate" days in our example and you will be using 90% of your "heavy" day MTL:

405 x 0.9 = 365lbs

This means you will squat 5 sets of 4 reps with 365lbs. If you were able to complete all the sets and reps in our Squat example your following workouts should look like this: Monday – 5x2 (415lbs)

Friday – 5x6 (332lbs)

Wednesday – 5x4 (374lbs)

Similarly to other phases, the first week or two of using ATP should be allotted to "easing" into training. These initial few training sessions could be carried out in a straight *linear progression*, without cycling. For example, if an athlete is planning to use 405lbs for the first "heavy" squat workout, then the first two weeks could look like this: Monday #1 – 5x2 (315lbs)

Friday #1 – 5x2 (355lbs)

Wednesday #2 – 5x2 (385lbs)

And only starting from week #3 this athlete would start using cycling schemes: Monday #3 – 5x2 (405lbs)

Friday #3 – 5x6 (324lbs)

Wednesday #4 – 5x4 (365lbs)

Monday #5 – 5x2 (415lbs)

During "light" and "moderate" days the weight will feel pretty comfortable, but this doesn't mean that you get to relax. Good work done on these days will insure successful performance on the following 5x2 day, so make every rep count. Lift the weight as fast as possible during all work sets (approach called *compensatory acceleration training*). Such explosive style, however, is not an excuse for sloppy form. Only the speed of ascent should increase. All other technical components of exercise execution stay the same.

Not every gym has sets of the very small plates available. Therefore, using exact weights from your calculation might not be possible. No worries. Just round the products of your calculations to the closest weight you can construct. For example, 324 could be rounded to 325. 353 could be rounded to either 352.5 or 355.

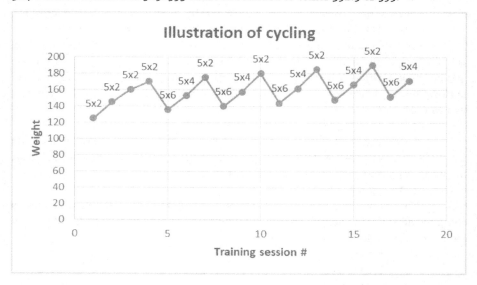

It is generally recommended that deadlifts are to be scheduled only once a week. In ATP every exercise is performed three times in two weeks. This should not be a problem since only one of those three training sessions is designated to be heavy. Still, however, if you deadlift substantial loads you might start developing some tension in your lower back.

Possible solution here is to perform only 3 or fewer work sets in deadlift instead of five. This goes for heavy, moderate and light days. You could also gradually decrease the number of sets as the weight increases. For example, if you are planning a 12 week ATP cycle you will do five sets during the first 4 weeks, four sets during weeks 5-8, and three sets during weeks 9-12. Experiment with using 85% and 70% for moderate and light days respectively for deadlift (or any other exercise for that matter) if recovery remains an issue.

Since in dips the weight of an athlete is the big component of the total load used, the calculations of the MTLs need to be adjusted when you figuring out 90% and 80% from the weight assigned as 100%. In the formula presented below I estimate that about 85% of the athlete's bodyweight is part of the total load in this exercise (in addition to MTL used by hanging a dumbbell, for example). Therefore, when deciding MTLs for dips on Friday-A/Wednesday-A, the following equation should be used:

$$MTL_{R\%} = R\% \times \frac{(0.85Q + Z)}{100\%} - 0.85Q$$

$MTL_{R\%}$ – load used in addition to the weight of an athlete;

$R\%$ - percentage of the MTL assigned for that training session;

Q – weight of an athlete;

Z – MTL used as 100% for that microcycle (on Monday-A).

This formula does not work unless you are able to use additional weight of at least 20-25% of your bodyweight on the "heavy" dips day. Until then perform dips in hypertrophy mode. This modification could also be applied to barbell bent-over rows to reduce the overall training stress. This way instead of using three stage microcycle, in these two exercises you will do 3 sets of 12-8 reps.

At some point the loads could become so great that performing three exercises in one session is no longer practical. In this case you can drop the last exercise of each training session and focus on four lifts only. At this time you could also start doing shoulder presses in the beginning of the B training session. The reason here is that eventually deadlifts will become so taxing that you will be too wiped out to stay productive for the following shoulder press.

Odd Weeks

MONDAY - A	WEDNESDAY - B	FRIDAY - A
Barbell bench press 5x2 (100%)	Standing barbell military press 5x4 (90%)	Barbell bench press 5x6 (80%)
Back squat 5x2 (100%)	Deadlift 5x4 (90%)	Back squat 5x6 (80%)

Even Weeks

MONDAY - B	WEDNESDAY - A	FRIDAY - B
Standing barbell military press 5x2 (100%)	Barbell bench press 5x4 (90%)	Standing barbell military press 5x6 (80%)
Deadlift 5x2 (100%)	Back squat 5x4 (90%)	Deadlift 5x6 (80%)

These abbreviated exercise complexes also land themselves nicely for another training method that might be appropriate for advanced athletes. At some point, regardless of how diligent you are about training and recovery, your body just "falls asleep" and stops responding. It needs a kick in the butt to wake up and high rep sets of squats and deadlift are just what the doctor ordered.

We are talking about an old shock technique called *widowmaker* that seems to be forgotten these days. It entails performing of just one heavy set of twenty reps in either squat or deadlift. The thinking is that such concentrated intense effort forces the body into immediate adaptation.

Realistically estimate the weight you could start with for twenty reps and then back down some more. As far as the bench and standing presses, you can stay with 5x6/5x4/5x2 wave or utilize straight linear progression in 5x5 scheme.

Obviously, this approach will also require close monitoring of the recovery. Even with your best effort in that area, however, you might still need to reduce frequency of training as the cycle progresses. For example, instead of three weekly sessions you might switch to training once every three days. Some might also go as far as training twice a week towards the end of a cycle:

MONDAY - A	FRIDAY - B
Barbell bench press 5x5	Standing barbell military press 5x5
Back squat 1x20	Deadlift 1x20

Even with these adjustments it is unlikely that you will be able to sustain such beating for too long. Don't be a hero and monitor yourself for signs of overtraining (decreased performance, loss of motivation, persistent feeling of fatigue, etc.). Get all you can out of the phase and switch to something more conventional. Odds are you won't be looking forward to getting back to this style of training any time soon.

Advanced training program 2

The training program presented here utilizes *conjugate sequence periodization* model and is strictly for the very elite portion of the gym population. If you are not quite in this category, you can still read it for informative purposes. This program is geared towards powerlifting but could also produce a significant increase of muscle mass. It is extremely challenging and a few things have to be considered before committing to it.

First and foremost, make sure you really need the level of training that is this demanding. It means that you have exhausted every other approach presented until this point. That should take you at least five years. If you are still making solid progress at the gym, there is no need to dive into any extremes. As Ronnie Coleman often said: "if it ain't broke, don't fix it."

Some might argue that this program is playing with fire for a drug free athlete. But this is the inevitable reality of training at the advanced level. Squatting 600 pounds is playing with fire. Benching 400 is playing with fire. *The closer you are to the limits of your genetic potential the more vigorous (and inherently dangerous) the training will have to become.*

This is a calculated risk elite athletes have to take in order to keep improving. At some point on order to make further progress you will almost inevitably have to overreach. The trick is to be able to balance it out accordingly with unloading periods, as the line between progressive overload and overtraining will become very-very thin.

On the other hand, there is no logical reason for beginners or intermediates to use ATP2 (or any other sophisticated techniques such as plyometrics, for example). Wear and tear accumulated from premature utilization of such methods could prevent them from ever reaching their highest possible levels of performance.

Assess your "energy budget" and decide if this program is a good fit for you at the moment. You will see that ATP2 takes exactly opposite direction from the training approach discussed at the end of the previous section. This program will definitely push the limits of recovery capability of a drug free athlete. Food and sleep have to be on point for the whole two months period. You should also consider if you simply have this much time to devote to training. For that reason I recommend to utilize weekends as much as possible.

Just like the rest of the "Big and Strong" training system, this program will be based on alteration of high volume and high intensity blocks of training. We will change the names of these blocks in order to use terminology that is more appropriate. Instead of hypertrophy phases, high volume blocks will be referred to as accumulation phases. Instead of strength phases, high intensity blocks will be referred to as realization phases.

The purpose of the accumulation phase is to shock the body with an increased workload (*concentrated loading* method). An athlete then gets a week of deload to allow fatigue to dissipate. As the recovery process is happening, the body is expected to increase fitness in order to adapt to the demand placed on it. At this time (during realization phase) an athlete will attempt progressively heavier loads in order to collect on the investment he made during accumulation phase.

Usually, as hypertrophy and strength phases progress an athlete is moving towards using higher MTLs. Things will flow slightly differently in ATP2. During accumulation phase the volume will be increasing from week to week while the loads are kept constant. During the realization phase the volume will be decreasing and the loads are expected to go up.

You will use your own judgment when deciding the intensity and volume for the deload weeks. Very advanced athletes should be able to estimate precise ranges based on their experience. If you purposely plan conservative intensity level for the accumulation phase, both deload weeks could be omitted. In this case it might be a good idea to switch to Monday, Wednesday, Friday, Saturday training schedule during accumulation phase in order to create two days of rest before the beginning of realization phase. If, on the other hand, the phase ends up being very taxing, only two training sessions for the following deload week might be warranted. This week is also a good time to step up active recovery procedures such as massage, contrast shower and some easy stretching.

Week 1 (deload/introductory)

TUESDAY	THURSDAY	SATURDAY
Back squat	Standing barbell military press	Back squat
Barbell bench press	Deadlift	Barbell bench press

Accumulation phase

During this phase we will be using a portion of an old training cycling model designed by USSR weightlifting coach Aleksey Medvedev. For all three weeks MTL for a particular exercise will stay the same. As the phase progresses the reps will be increasing on Saturday and Sunday sessions. The volume on Tuesdays and Thursdays will be kept the same and they will be considered active rest days. Take that into account when you are programming loads for deficit halting deadlifts and rack pulls.

One could also consider performing some of the exercises on Tuesdays and Thursdays in Westside Barbell style speed mode (*dynamic effort*). In this case chains or elastic bands could be utilized but the load would have to be reduced (MTLs for the same exercise would be different on Tuesday/Thursday and Saturday/Sunday). One exercise for upper body and one exercise for lower body should be more than enough. Also, keep in mind that these days should still stay relatively easy.

Week 2

TUESDAY	THURSDAY	SATURDAY	SUNDAY
Back squat 6x3	Standing barbell military press 6x3	Back squat 6x4	Standing barbell military press 6x4
Barbell bench press 6x3	Deficit halting deadlift 6x3*	Barbell bench press 6x4	Deadlift 6x4
Front squat 6x3	Close grip barbell bench press 6x3	Front squat 6x4	Close grip barbell bench press 6x4
Dip 6x3	Rack pull 6x3**	Dip 6x4	Barbell bent-over row 6x4

Week 3

TUESDAY	THURSDAY	SATURDAY	SUNDAY
Back squat 6x3	Standing barbell military press 6x3	Back squat 6x5	Standing barbell military press 6x5
Barbell bench press 6x3	Deficit halting deadlift 6x3*	Barbell bench press 6x5	Deadlift 6x5
Front squat 6x3	Close grip barbell bench press 6x3	Front squat 6x5	Close grip barbell bench press 6x5
Dip 6x3	Rack pull 6x3**	Dip 6x5	Barbell bent-over row 6x5

Week 4

TUESDAY	THURSDAY	SATURDAY	SUNDAY
Back squat 6x3	Standing barbell military press 6x3	Back squat 6x6	Standing barbell military press 6x6
Barbell bench press 6x3	Deficit halting deadlift 6x3*	Barbell bench press 6x6	Deadlift 6x6
Front squat 6x3	Close grip barbell bench press 6x3	Front squat 6x6	Close grip barbell bench press 6x6
Dip 6x3	Rack pull 6x3**	Dip 6x6	Barbell bent-over row 6x6

* Deadlift performed to the knee level while standing on a 2 inch block
** Deadlift performed in the power rack or off the blocks with barbell starting position set up at the knee level

When you are deciding on MTL for a particular exercise, think about what it is going to feel like on the Saturday/Sunday of week 4. You want those days to be very challenging, but still to be able to complete all sets and reps without going to a total failure. Most of it will fall around 70% of 1RM, but that's just an estimate. Even though you will be using sets across schemes, feel free to increase or decrease the weight by 10-20 pounds on those days depending on how it goes. Keep in mind that it is not about performance in any individual exercise, but about cumulative fatigue the phase is designed to create.

Realization phase

Do not get overzealous right from the start of the realization phase. It is possible that you will still be recuperating from the accumulation phase in the first week or two. As a result, when you work your way up to 5RMs the weight might feel heavier than expected. On the other hand, smaller athletes might feel fully recovered and ready for new PRs. In either case, pushing the issue at this point could sabotage the whole training cycle. Therefore, it might be better to look at 5RM training session as a data collection point to see where you stand. This information will help you more accurately estimate loads for 3RM and 1RM workouts.

Since this program is designed to be used only by very experienced athletes, we can now utilize the Borg ratings of perceived exertion (RPE) scale. This scale measures the difficulty of physical activity on the scale from 6 (no exertion) to 20 (maximum exertion). If you don't find such guidance useful, simply look at Tuesday sessions as moderate, Thursday sessions as light and Saturday sessions as heavy.

Not all heavy days will be the same. Both 5RM and 3RM sessions should be carried out without excessive psychological arousal. During these sessions it is better to aim for the loads with which you have at least one repetition left in the tank (referred to as *buffer*) after completing prescribed reps. Only the Saturday of week eight should be an all-out war.

Week 5 (deload)

WEDNESDAY	SATURDAY
Back squat	Back squat
Barbell bench press	Barbell bench press
Barbell bent-over row	Deadlift

Week 6

TUESDAY (12 RPE)	THURSDAY (10 RPE)	SATURDAY (16 RPE)
Front squat 5x5	Standing barbell military press 3X12-8	Back squat 5RM
Close grip barbell bench press 5x5	Pull-up 3x12-8	Barbell bench press 5RM
Barbell bent-over row 5x5	Dip 3x12-8	Deadlift 5RM

Week 7

TUESDAY (13 RPE)	THURSDAY (11 RPE)	SATURDAY (18 RPE)
Front squat 4x5	Standing barbell military press 2X12-8	Back squat 3RM
Close grip barbell bench press 4x5	Pull-up 2x12-8	Barbell bench press 3RM
Barbell bent-over row 4x5	Dip 2x12-8	Deadlift 3RM

Week 8

TUESDAY (14 RPE)	THURSDAY (12 RPE)	SATURDAY or SUNDAY (20 RPE)
Front squat 3x5	Standing barbell military press 1X12-8	Back squat 1RM
Close grip barbell bench press 3x5	Pull-up 1x12-8	Barbell bench press 1RM
Barbell bent-over row 3x5	Dip 1x12-8	Deadlift 1RM

As was stated earlier in this book, programming for advanced athletes becomes highly individualized. There are simply too many variables at this level. What works for 405 bench might not work for 455, and what works for 455 might not work for 495. ATP2 is just an example of how training could be planned. Experience and knowledge of an athlete will be determining the precise recommendation.

One of the main concerns at the advanced level for a drug free trainee is that simultaneous improvement of multiple athletic qualities becomes increasingly difficult. For example, beginners might not have any problem working on increasing squat and distance running at the same time, but advanced athletes no longer have such luxury. This makes block periodization the only sustainable way to keep progressing at the highest level. The trick is to schedule these blocks in the manner that allows maximum transformation of performance gains from one phase to another (approach called *phase potentiation*). "Periodization: Theory and Methodology of Training" explains how various training modes should be properly sequenced.

Another factor that has to be taken into account at this level is that peak performance cannot be maintained for extended periods of time. For example, it is not unusual to see novices trying to break new 1RM in bench press almost every time they are at the gym. Although this is not the smartest thing to do, nothing dramatic usually happens. But can you imagine that international level powerlifter was doing the same thing? An injury or overtraining would be right around the corner. Pushing your body to an absolute limit should not be attempted frequently. This implies that advanced training unavoidably has to be cyclical. Think of it as if you were trying to jump over a wide ditch. Most likely you would take a few steps back first.

Weightlifting

I would like to start this section by the word of caution. Classic Olympic lifts are very complex and should not be self-taught. Adequate description of their techniques and learning methods would almost double the size of this book. If you don't have a serious trainer (your online "coach" doesn't count) to help you master these movement, it is better to leave them alone. Also, due to high skill component in weightlifting competitive lifts have to be practiced more often. This means that all the additional exercises have to be carefully planned to make sure overall workload does not exceed the recovery capacity.

Week 1

MONDAY – A	WEDNESDAY – B	FRIDAY – C
Snatch 1RM	Clean and jerk 3x1 (95%)	Snatch 5x1 (90%)
Standing barbell military press 5x2	Back squat 5x4	Deadlift 5x6

Week 2

MONDAY – D	WEDNESDAY – A	FRIDAY – B
Clean and jerk 1RM	Snatch 3x1 (95%)	Clean and jerk 5x1 (90%)
Front squat 5x2	Standing barbell military press 5x4	Back squat 5x6

Week 3

MONDAY – C	WEDNESDAY – D	FRIDAY – A
Snatch 1RM	Clean and jerk 3x1 (95%)	Snatch 5x1 (90%)
Deadlift 5x2	Front squat 5x4	Standing barbell military press 5x6

Week 4

MONDAY – B	WEDNESDAY – C	FRIDAY – D
Clean and jerk 1RM	Snatch 3x1 (95%)	Clean and jerk 5x1 (90%)
Back squat 5x2	Deadlift 5x4	Front squat 5x6

The overall structure of this program might appear complicated at first. If you find this a bit confusing, simply follow the program as it is presented in the tables until you start to recognize the patterns. You will basically use a three stage microcycle format similar to the one in ATP: heavy day, moderate day and light day. What these days actually mean will differ for classic lifts (snatch and clean and jerk) and assistance exercises (which weightlifters consider everything that is not a classic lift).

The microcycle for the classic lifts will begin on Monday with working up to a 1 RM for either of the exercises. This does not mean that you literally have to attempt an all-time PR on every 1RM day. These weights could be preplanned for the whole training period with a scheduled peak at the end. For example:

205 for week 1,
210 for week 3,
215 for week 5,
etc.

Work your way up with small increments, even if it takes you 10 or more sets. Power snatches and power cleans could be performed as the first few warm ups before switching to full snatches or cleans. Don't try to save your energy by cutting down on warm up. Remember, classic lifts are as much about technical proficiency as they are about strength. Therefore, use these lighter sets to sharpen your form.

If you missed a lift due to technical error but felt that you should've had it, back down 20-30 pounds and work your way up again. If the weight is missed again use the highest one you were successful with for all calculations for this microcycle.

Let's say you successfully lifted 200 pounds in snatch on Monday, The next time you will do this lift will be on Friday and it will be a light day. Calculate 90% of your current 1RM (200 x 0.9 = 180) and perform 5 singles with it. The next Wednesday is a moderate day for that lift. Calculate 95% if your current 1RM (200 x .95 = 190) and perform 3 singles with it. Monday of week three is a new 1RM day for snatch. You will attempt a slightly heavier weight and, if successful, will adjust your calculations for the following two sessions in snatch accordingly.

Once you are done with the classic lift of the session, you will move on to the assistance exercise (press, squat, deadlift and front squat). These will be performed with your basic ATP wave, described in the respective section. However, since we are rotating four different complexes here, the order of light, moderate and heavy days for each particular exercise will be 5X2/5x4/5x6. What stays the same is that you always calculate your light and moderate days based on the last 5x2 weight.

Once the main part of the session is completed, LIMITED amount of accessory work could be added. These would be exercises directed to address any lagging portions of either of the classic lifts. They should not be a constant part of the training process and can vary over time depending on the needs. If, however, your particular situation requires some additional exercises on the regular basis, there is a logical way to arrange it.

For example, if you want to add some work in jerk behind the neck from the blocks, it could be planned in the following manner. On your 5x2 days (regardless of in which exercise) you could add 3 sets of 3reps in this exercise (excluding warm-ups) after the main two lifts are completed. On the following 5x4 days you will do 2 sets of 3 reps, and on 5x6 day you will do one set of 3 reps. This way you would create a mini taper within a week before each 1RM day of the following week.

Obviously this is just one example and it doesn't even have to be this complicated. The main thing to remember is that *any additional work should be there for a specific reason* and not because you have time to kill. "The Weightlifting Encyclopedia" goes over many assistance exercises and their purpose.

Based on your experience level, this program can be squeezed into four or more weekly sessions. You just have to follow the order of the prescribed workouts. That means that light, moderate and heavy sessions will not fall on the same days of the week:

Week 1

MONDAY – A	TUESDAY – B	THURSDAY – C	SATURDAY – D
Snatch 1RM	Clean and jerk 3X1 (95%)	Snatch 5X1 (90%)	Clean and jerk 1RM
Standing barbell military press 5x2	Back squat 5x4	Deadlift 5x6	Front squat 5x2

Week 2

MONDAY – A	TUESDAY – B	THURSDAY – C	SATURDAY – D
Snatch 3x1 (95%)	Clean and jerk 5x1 (90%)	Snatch 1RM	Clean and jerk 3x1 (95%)
Standing barbell military press 5x4	Back squat 5x6	Deadlift 5x2	Front squat 5x4

Week 3

MONDAY – A	TUESDAY or WEDNESDAY – B	THURSDAY – C	SATURDAY – D
Snatch 5x1 (90%)	Clean and jerk 1RM	Snatch 3x1 (95%)	Clean and jerk 5x1 (90%)
Standing barbell military press 5x6	Back squat 5x2	Deadlift 5x4	Front squat 5x6

The number of weekly sessions could be varied strategically. For example, you could train 4 times a week for a few weeks (preparatory phase) while not attempting the heaviest loads. Later the number of weekly sessions could be reduced to 3 (competitive phase) but with heavier weights. You could also increase contrast between these phases by adding considerable amount of ancillary exercises during preparatory phase and then removing them completely in the competitive phase. If even narrower specialization is sought after in the competitive phase, an athlete could switch to the "Bulgarian" version of this program:

Odd weeks

MONDAY – A	WEDNESDAY – B	FRIDAY – A
Snatch 1RM	Clean and jerk 3x1 (95%)	Snatch 5x1 (90%)
Front squat 5x2	Back squat 5x4	Front squat 5x6

Even weeks

MONDAY – B	WEDNESDAY – A	FRIDAY – B
Clean and jerk 1RM	Snatch 3x1 (95%)	Clean and jerk 5x1 (90%)
Back squat 5x2	Front squat 5x4	Back squat 5x6

Conditioning

The material we have covered so far was focused exclusively on getting bigger and stronger. I do realize, however, that this is not a priority for everyone. Large portion of the gym population just wants to get physically fit and lose some fat in the process. Such goal does not imply that your workout should consist of wandering from one machine to another while mostly looking at the phone. It also doesn't mean that you have to flip tires or hop around the gym.

The program presented here is designed to turn you into a well-rounded athlete and make you look like one. It is essentially CrossFit style of training, minus all the craziness. Every training session will target multiple energy systems. If you don't have any experience with this style of training, start very-very easy.

Odd Weeks

MONDAY – 1A	WEDNESDAY – 1B	FRIDAY – 1C
Back squat 5x5	Barbell bench press 5x5	Deadlift 5x5
CIRCUIT: 1. Pulldown 5x10 2. Standing dumbbell press 5x10 3. Lunge 5x(5+5)	CIRCUIT: 1.Seated cable row 5x10 2. Dumbbell bench press 5x10 3. Goblet squat 5x10	CIRCUIT: 1. Pulldown 5x10 2. Standing dumbbell press 5x10 3. Lunge 5x(5+5)
Back extension 1xAMRAP	Incline sit-up 1xAMRAP	Back extension 1xAMRAP
Treadmill 3x3 min	Treadmill 4x3 min	Treadmill 5x3 min

Even weeks

MONDAY – 2A	WEDNESDAY – 2B	FRIDAY – 2C
Back squat 5x5	Barbell bench press 5x5	Deadlift 5x5
CIRCUIT: 1.Seated cable row 5x10 2. Dumbbell bench press 5x10 3. Goblet squat 5x10	CIRCUIT: 1. Pulldown 5x10 2. Standing dumbbell press 5x10 3. Lunge 5x(5+5)	CIRCUIT: 1.Seated cable row 5x10 2. Dumbbell bench press 5x10 3. Goblet squat 5x10
Incline sit-up 1xAMRAP	Back extension 1xAMRAP	Incline sit-up 1xAMRAP
Treadmill 3x3 min	Treadmill 4x3 min	Treadmill 5x3 min

The first exercise of the session will be performed for 5 sets of 5 reps (not counting the warm-ups). I recommend that you start at about 80-90% of what you would normally use for 5x5 in each exercise, and then see how it goes. Just keep in mind that you won't be able to increase the weight from session to session at the same rate as in other training phases. This is because you will be spreading your "energy budget" over wider range of athletic qualities.

The more advanced athletes can also utilize 5X6/5X4/5X2 microcycle for these exercises, as explained in the ATP section. The difference here will be that the whole microcycle will take three weeks. First week you will do 5x6 in all strength exercises, second week 5x4 and the third week 5x2. Cyclical variations of intensity and volume could be also implement for the remaining portion of the workout.

The first exercise will be the most "relaxed" part of the session, since you get to rest 2 to 3 minutes between each set. After you are done with the strength movement, you will move on to a circuit rotation. These are designed in such way that there should be a minimum time for transitioning from one exercise to the next, even in a crowded gym. Once you are done with shoulder presses, for example, you will drop dumbbells to your sides and immediately proceed to lunges with the same dumbbells (five lunges on each leg).

Similarly, during your next session, after you finish first set of **seated cable rows**, you will grab a pair of dumbbells (probably slightly heavier than you used for shoulder presses) and lay down on the same bench you were just sitting on while rowing. Once you complete dumbbell bench presses, you will put one of the dumbbells to a side and move on to the goblet squats while holding the other dumbbell by your chest with two hands. After that, you put the dumbbell down and go back to the horizontal rows right away.

As you can see, that's three exercises performed for five sets of ten reps with absolutely zero rest in between. This should make it obvious that the weights you will use here shouldn't be even close to your 10 rep maxes in those exercises. Therefore, don't be too greedy with the weight reduction. Get used to this pace first and then start slowly increasing the weights you are using from session to session.

Slightly easier way to perform the circuits would be by utilizing every minute on the minute (EMOM) protocol. This way you perform one set of an exercise in the beginning of every minute. Once all the prescribed reps are completed, you will rest the remaining time of that minute before moving on to the following exercise.

Your heart rate will be racing after the circuits are completed. To get little break before the cardio, you will rest a minute or two and perform a set of either back extensions or sit-ups. In each exercise you will do as many reps as possible (AMRAP) and then try to beat that number by at least one rep at the next session. If you can do many more than 20 reps, add a little more resistance at the next session. Grab a plate and hold it over your chest with your arms crossed.

Once again, rest for a minute or two and we are off to cardio. I prefer to use the treadmill because it is easier to control all the parameters. We will be using 3 to 1 ratio. That means you will run for three minutes and then walk for one. On Monday you will do three rounds like that, on Wednesday – 4, and on Friday – 5.

If you started with 5 mph and have gone through all three sessions, you will increase the speed by 0.1 mph and go back to 3x3, 4x3 and 5x3. When that's accomplished you'll go up to 5.2 and go through rotation again. If you were unable to complete all prescribed rounds, you will stay with the same speed for the next week.

It will take some experimentation to find what speed is comfortable for you to start with. As always, it is better to start too easy than too hard. If you feel that you underestimated your endurance and the first week was way too easy, try 0.2 speed increase for the next week. For the minute long active rest periods between the rounds you will use comfortable walking speed. Somewhere around 3 mph. This speed stays constant throughout.

Once running is completed, add some stretching and you are done for the day. It might not appear all that challenging at first, but little by little the weights you are using in circuits and the speed on the treadmill will go up. In just a few weeks this program will be testing your mental fortitude. Even if you train primarily for muscle size and strength, it might still be beneficial to *include this program periodically as general physical preparation (GPP) phases to improve workload capacity and recovery capabilities.*

If this program is being used as part of preparation for an athletic event (MMA match, for example), some modification could be implemented. Strength exercises could be substituted with more explosive lifts closer to the competition. Thrusters alternated with power cleans and push presses are your best options.

The power movements do not necessarily have to be performed in sets across scheme. Instead you could just start with some easy fives and work your way up to heavier loads. For example, for the first 2–3 weeks you would work up to triples, the next 2–3 weeks – to doubles and the last 2–3 weeks of preparation – to singles. Depending on the size of an athlete, all strength and conditioning work will stop a week or two away from competition and the focus will shift to the sport specific training.

Another way to make this program more athletic would be by adding LIMITED amount of explosive drills once the strength exercises are completed (before proceeding with the circuits). The idea is similar to the *complex training*, where heavy resistance exercises are used as warm-up for the nervous system before performing power movements. For example, an athlete could perform some short sprints after completing all work sets of squats, a few sets of medicine ball throws after bench press and some box jumps after deadlifts.

On the other hand, for a beginner level trainee modifications will be in the direction of making the program easier. For example, instead of performing circuits, all exercises could performed in straight fashion (completing all sets in one exercise before moving to the next). Significantly overweight trainees could also initially use walking (while slowly increasing the distance) instead of running.

NUTRITION

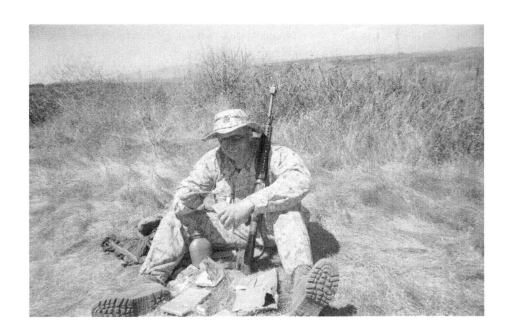

"Get comfortable being uncomfortable."
\- Jillian Michaels

There is a lot of confusion on this topic and l will try not to add to it. Seems that common sense becomes less and less common when it comes to nutrition. In theory we could calculate how many grams of each macronutrient we need. Make sure everything is organic and gluten free. Plus don't forget about eliminating all the bad cholesterol, of course. In reality, however, there are too many individual variables that have to be taken into account. Therefore, it is difficult to provide any guidelines specific enough to be useful.

The more practical approach is to take your current diet and try to improve it over time. Making small changes is the key here. Anything too radical will most likely not last very long. Monitor your appearance in the mirror and your performance in the gym while you are manipulating your diet. *If you use "Big and Strong" system as prescribed and still not gaining weight, most likely you are not eating or sleeping enough.*

Meal schedule

Let's start with the meal schedule. Ideally you should be eating 4-6 times a day with your meals evenly spread out. Generally, the smaller and leaner your meals are the more of them you will be able to squeeze in one day (large fatty meals will sit in your stomach longer). **Also, try not lie down right after meals. Instead take a short walk to expedite the emptying of the stomach.**

If you currently eat three times a day, try to have a snack somewhere. It is really not that hard and a very busy schedule is no excuse. For instance, if there is a long gap between your breakfast and lunch, just add an apple and a handful of almonds somewhere in between. Don't change too many things at once and give your body time to adjust. You can't go overnight from eating three times a day to eating eight. Just like you can't jump from squatting 300 pounds to squatting 800.

We all know that breakfast is the most important meal. It fuels you for the rest of the day. There is one more important meal though. It is thought that immediately after training sessions our metabolism is in its heightened state and the ability of muscle tissue to uptake nutrients is increased. This window is considered to be open for about an hour and it would be wise to have a quality meal within this time.

One more thing you have to take into account when spacing your meals throughout the day is your pre workout meal timing. A lot of it is a matter of personal preference. In general after a large meal you should allow about three hours before hitting the gym. After medium size meal two hours and after small size meal about an hour. Try to avoid anything with a lot of fat or fiber at this time as this will slow the digestion and might make you feel bloated during the following training session.

Calories

Calories are used to measure the amount of energy we receive from consuming one gram of a *macronutrient*. The latter includes protein, carbohydrates (carbs) and fats. One gram of protein or carbs has 4 calories. One gram of fat has 9. Such difference in energy density is one of the reasons to keep consumption of fats under control when dieting (unless you selected increasingly popular "ketogenic" rout).

Protein

Besides feeding yourself consistently throughout the day make sure to get some protein with every meal. Amino acids derived from protein are considered to be the primary medium for muscle tissue synthesis. Therefore, you want to have at least some amount of them circulating in your bloodstream at all times. Best sources are eggs, beef, pork, milk (if tolerated), chicken and fish. If the budget allows, you can utilize protein supplements. Don't think of them as a magic pill. They are just convenient to use sometimes. For example, if your gym is far from your house and you are unable to have a meal within an hour after your workout, protein shake could be an answer.

Carbs

Carb overview will be a little more extensive. Not because they are more important than other macronutrients, but because few basic concepts need to be understood in their regard. As always, we will simplify things a little and this quick overview is not meant to turn you into registered dietitian.

Carbs are your primary fuel source. Once a meal rich in carbs has been consumed, they are broken down and absorbed into a blood stream as glucose. The rate at which this process occurs depends on the type of carbs your meal contains. In general all carbohydrates can be roughly divided into fast absorption (simple) carbs and slow absorption (complex) carbs. Term Glycemic Index (GI) is also commonly used. The higher GI is the faster the absorption will occur. That means that simple carbs have high GI and complex carbs have low GI.

Our bodies always try to maintain certain steady concentration of glucose in the blood. If the blood glucose levels were allowed to drop very low, there wouldn't be an energy source readily available for utilization. If the levels were allowed to raise too high, the blood would start to resemble a maple syrup which would impede circulation.

We are now going to take a look at what happens when you consume a meal full of simple carbs (candy, soda, pastries, etc.) versus meal consisting of mostly complex carbs (pasta, rice, potatoes, oatmeal and yams). Let's say one day you decided to have some donuts and soda for breakfast (point A).

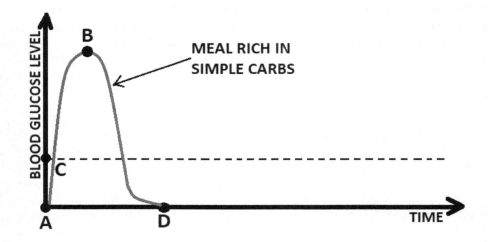

Since your breakfast choices consist of mostly simple carbs, they will be absorbed very quickly and result a steep increase of the blood glucose level (point B). This will trigger significant release of insulin in order to bring blood glucose level down to a desirable level (dotted line C). All excess sugar will be removed from circulation and stored away as body fat to be utilized later.

Depending on the size of your breakfast, all this might happen in an hour or two. But now let's imagine that you have 4 hours between breakfast and lunch (point D). Where are you going to get the energy for the other two hours? Those who have been paying attention so far will answer: from stored body fat. That is partially correct answer. Good job! Bear in mind, however, that when our body is in starvation mode it will also tap into muscle tissue as a source of energy. Such catabolic process is obviously not desirable. Also, since you will be you essentially fasting from at this point, feeling of low energy and fatigue will accompany that time period.

The situation will be different if you eat bowl of oatmeal for breakfast. Oatmeal is a complex carb and will be digested slowly. This means that you will have a steady source of energy for longer. It also means that you will avoid storing of body fat (when blood glucose is too high) and tapping into muscle tissues for energy (when blood glucose is too low).

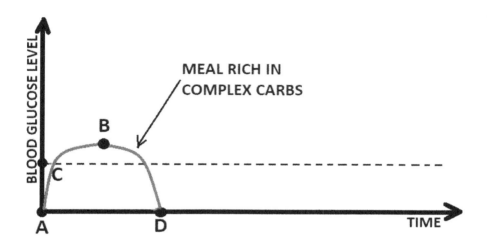

Hopefully the above comparison of how different types of carbs get utilized made it clear that any extreme fluctuations of blood glucose level are undesirable. For that reason it is also generally recommended that instead of large seldom meals, athletes consume smaller but more frequent meals (A, B, C, D, E). Such eating practice will also give you chance to maintain steady intake of protein throughout the day.

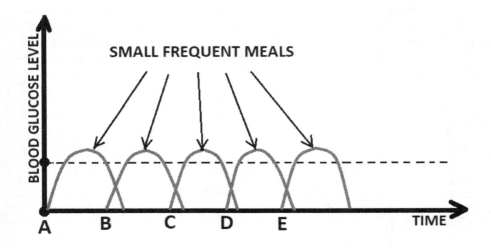

Carb consumption differs from the protein though. When it comes to protein you generally want to keep its intake even throughout the day. With carbs, on the other hand, try to get more of them earlier in the day and gradually decrease their consumption as the day goes on. This is due to the fact that carbs consumed later in the day will have smaller chance if being utilized for energy and higher chance of being store as fat (some of it will be absorbed when you are already in bed). To illustrate, have eggs with large portion of oatmeal for breakfast, steak with moderate amount of potatoes for lunch and chicken with small amount of rice for dinner. Your late evening snack could be completely carb free. Cottage cheese or greek yogurt could do the trick.

There are two exceptions here. Both pre and post workout meals should contain carbs combined with some protein in it. Even if you train late in the evening. Immediately after training session is also the time when you can get away with eating some of your simple carbs (sports drink, for example) to jumpstart the recovery process. Due to prolonged fasting at night, you can also have some simple carbs (combined with predominantly complex carbs) with breakfast. At other times try to stay away from simple carbs. Soda and other sugary drinks are the frequent offenders in this category.

Fats

When it comes to fat you don't need to worry about getting enough of it. Most of common diets will provide fat in excess. Therefore, your effort should be directed towards keeping the amount of fat consumed under control. Once again, common sense applies. Reduction of fats below reasonable level is not only unnecessary but is also unhealthy. If your diet is full of junk food (pizza, fries, chips), you have some work to do. But as long as you stick to the staple foods mentioned earlier for the most of your meals, you should be on the right track.

Fiber

Most of us have an idea of what eating healthy means. Eating lots of fresh fruits and vegetables is always a good policy. Besides being rich in *micronutrients* (vitamins and minerals), fruits and vegetables are an important source of fiber. One of the many benefits of dietary fiber is that it makes your gastrointestinal tract work more efficiently. This is a huge aid when you are trying to get enough nutrients while trying to recover from grueling training sessions. As always, there is no need for anything extreme. Putting away massive amounts of broccoli and asparagus every day will not make you live forever. Instead it will fill your belly with gas and discomfort.

Water

Water is not considered to be a nutrient but we might as well cover its intake here. Among the factors that will determine the exact amount you need are your local climate, activity level, etc. Simple way to monitor your hydration status is to check the color of your urine. If it's dark and brown start drinking more. Besides drinking with meals, good times to add more water are upon awakening, half hour before meals and before/during/after training sessions. Don't dive at the deep end right away. Start adding little by little and keep watching the color of your urine. Once it consistently has clear yellowish color you know you found the right amount of water you need.

Supplements

As far as dietary supplements your budget will be the determining factor. Start with basics. I mentioned protein powder earlier. Also, taking multivitamins and multiminerals with breakfast is an easy way to make sure all your micronutrients are covered. Creatine is another proven supplement that has been around for some time. Just stick to the minimum recommended doses and be especially diligent about staying hydrated if you decide to take it. Aside from this short list, make sure to do research before spending money on a new "ultimate" pill endorsed by some celebrity athlete. The chances are that athlete has never taken it.

Weight loss

The purpose of this book is to help you get bigger and stronger. With today's obesity problem, however, I feel obligated to say at least a few words about losing weight. Everything we have discussed in this section so far will apply, whether you trying to gain muscle mass or lose body fat. The main difference is that *when the goal is to gain muscle you have to consume more calories than you spend and when the goal is to lose fat you have to consume less than you spend.*

On paper it sounds simple but in practice results will vary substantially. A fighter can lose 30-40 pounds in a month or two, while someone else is struggling to lose a pound. There are many possible reasons for it but here is an observation I have made over years: some people are obsessed with food. As they are eating one meal they are already thinking about the next one. The moment they go on a diet, they start craving everything. They are contemplating their cheat meals for days. They are constantly looking up healthy recipes and counting calories. They just can't stop thinking about food. They are ADDICTED.

Looking at this situation from such perspective explains why some people are repeatedly unsuccessful with losing weight: they never really address the main issue. For example, one of the mistakes people make while "dieting" is trying to enjoy the limited amount of food they are consuming as much as possible. This is an ill strategy because by doing so they surrender to the power of food over them. You can't win a fight over this addiction with such defeated mindset.

The more sound approach is to deal with this addiction as you would with alcoholism. Forget about losing weight and focus on cleansing your mind instead. Just like you would get rid of all the alcohol while trying to quit drinking, clean up your house of all the junk food. Get rid of all the spices while you are at it. Your food doesn't have to taste good. You don't need all the variety. You don't need a hidden stash of candy for "emergency" situations. You don't need your morning coffee to be ready for work. Eliminate these tantrums! Eliminate your weakness!

Once the house is clean, you are ready to get started. We are going to divide this process in two distinct steps. Do not attempt to accomplish both at the same time. Your first step is going to be to start eating clean. Decide on a few food items (preferably from the ones listed earlier in this chapter) that you allowed to have for the next few months. You can even go as far eating the same meal all day every day. Just make sure it has some protein and fiber in it. Adding multivitamin might be a good idea if you really limit your choices.

Do not try to restrict the amount of food you consume at this point. Once you learn eating clean, eating less will be a lot easier. Just stick to the same boring meal schedule without any attempt to starve yourself. Take a week or two to figure out how many meals and their sizes you need per day to feel comfortable. You can measure and record your food if it makes it easier. By then you should also realize why sticking to the limited number of food choices makes it easier to keep track of things.

Once you have been compliant for at least a week, you are ready for the second step. Slowly start reducing the portion sizes. Nothing too drastic. Just take away a little bit and stay with that for a week. If everything goes well, take away a little more next week. It shouldn't be too difficult concerning that you are probably sick of eating the same thing over and over again. At some point you will arrive at the amount of food that allows you to lose weight without feeling hungry. Hopefully your training will be coming along at the same time.

Things get much more complicated when you add social interaction to the equation. The unfortunate reality is that our current understanding of having fun still revolves around gathering together to eat a lot of unhealthy food. These events are normally accompanied by continuous meaningless conversations, therefore, at least some alcohol is recommended to get appropriate silly vibe.

Of course, it is unreasonable to recommend to stay away from all social functions, but do be aware that these situations will require significant restraint on your part. The problem is not that you will get fat overnight. The fact that you couldn't resist the temptation will remind you that you are still a slave of your addiction, which could leave you feeling disempowered and even depressed.

I am not suggesting that you should never enjoy food for the rest of your life. I am just saying that if obsession with food is suspected, temporary radical measures must be taken. There is no need to dance around this issue. For example, we don't say that it is okay to be a drug addict as long as you are happy. Think of it as food detox.

Once you defeat this addiction, start SLOWLY increasing the variety and tastefulness of your meals. It is important not to get inpatient at this time and jump right back to the old eating habits. Just like you wouldn't celebrate successful quitting of drinking by getting wasted, do not reward yourself for defeating food addiction by bingeing. If you do decide to treat yourself every once in a while, a good sign that you truly earned it if there is no feeling of shame afterwards.

Consistency

Just like with training, effective diet is all about consistence. Anyone can eat clean for a day or even a week. But what you think is going to happen when you return to your normal eating patterns? You are not the first person in the world who wants results as quickly as possible. If there was an easy way to get things done, it would be included in this book. It's not a conspiracy.

Abandon the mindset of a temporary fix and start moving towards developing the lifelong healthy eating habits. As I stated earlier, don't attempt to adjust your whole diet all at once. Instead try improving one meal at a time. Making sure you eat proper breakfast is always a good start. Once that's up to standards you can move on to the next step. When it comes to nutrition there is always room for improvement. Similarly to how your training will be more complex over time, your diet will have to become more refined as you keep advancing.

MOTIVATION

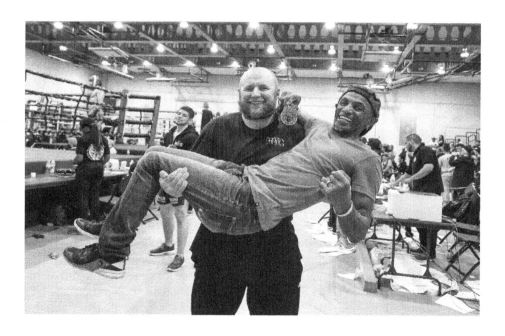

"We work jobs that we hate to buy things we don't need"
                                    – Quote from "Fight club" (modified)

Reading this section is completely optional. We will mostly be talking about the issues related to poor compliance with training. It always amazes me when grownups ask how I am able to stick to my training schedule. I am not even sure how to reply. I decided to do it and so I am doing it. If every training session and every meal gets me closer to whatever goal I have in mind, then why would there ever be struggle?

The bottom line is you don't have to workout if you don't want to. It is nobody's business what your midsection looks like. This book is not written for kids. I don't need to give a motivational speech that exercising and eating vegetables are good for you.

Sit down and write your personal priorities list on a piece of paper. Health, family and career will probably take the top spots. Whatever follows them is a personal choice. If things like PlayStation and watching football come before the gym, then don't even worry about it. Chances are you won't be able to follow through. Don't feel bad about it. Don't make excuses such as that you don't have time. It's just not something you really care about. Life goes on.

But if physical fitness scores high on your list and yet you are still not able to stick to the program, something else is going on. You probably lack basic DISCIPLINE. You don't get to control the weather. You don't get to control traffic. But what you should be able to control is yourself. Unfortunately discipline is no longer emphasized in our schools. Instead we teach our kids that having fun and being happy are the only important things in life. Well, by that logic eating ice-cream while watching Netflix is a lot more fun than doing burpees.

The outcomes of such upbringing are so systemic that now we make up excuses for our pathetic level of fitness on societal level. How about "bad genes" explanations for everything? Did our genetic makeup suddenly mutate over last few decades to explain skyrocketing of the obesity? Or how about the new notion of "curvy" models? It is interesting to see how sexy all this "curviness" is going to look when they are in their 40's. Not to mention the detrimental health consequences.

Don't fall for these lies. Don't use an excuse that you are "happy" with the way you are to cover up for your laziness. If there was a magic button that instantly gets you in shape, every single person would press it. If it were that easy, nobody would ever say that they actually prefer being weak and fat.

These days people are hyperaware of how they feel all the time. This is perhaps a consequence of enormous amount of reality television we are exposed to. If you spend a long enough time in front of a TV, it might appear that sitting down and talking about how we feel about all the aspects of our lives is a completely productive use of our time. Thus we start to analyze everything. For example, does going to the gym make me happy? Very few will answer this question with a resounding "yes."

But do we really need to look at everything this way? For example, do you wake up in the morning and start contemplating on how you feel about brushing your teeth today? How much fun do I have while doing it? Luckily we don't look at it this way. Brushing your teeth is something that a person does in the modern society. Wouldn't it be nice if people started looking at regular nonnegotiable exercising the same way? Just like some minimum level of hygiene and education are expected in our society, shouldn't there be a minimum acceptable level of fitness?

We have these amazing machines given to us at birth and we never bother with any maintenance. Would you do the same if you had a Ferrari? And would you always drive it in the first gear without ever exploring what this car is capable of? Well, this is what most of us do with our bodies.

People get drawn to comfort, but too much comfort could be destructive. Think of water in the fast mountain river. It is clean and full of energy. Now what about water in a puddle? It goes bad. Things grow in it. That puddle is you sitting on your behind while staring at your phone.

We don't really appreciate food unless we are hungry. We don't really appreciate our beds unless we are tired. It appears that we need at least some adversity to feel truly alive. Comfort is good but you have to earn it to truly enjoy it. You can do things like hunting or rock climbing to heighten your senses, but most of us are unable to schedule such adventures on a regular basis. Exercise is the easiest substitution.

A very common way for people to motivate themselves to exercise is by desire to be more appealing to the opposite sex. Most, however, realize pretty quickly that there are a lot easier ways to attract intimate partner. Guys become increasingly better at being masterful talking machines. Girls learn that a little bit of makeup goes a long way. And even all that goes out of the window once most of us get married. Such motivation is simply too superficial to encourage lifelong exercise habit.

Forget about all this nonsense. Forget about getting in shape for the summer. Forget about losing a few pounds to fit into a pretty dress. Make being physically fit a permanent part of who you are. You don't need to wait for the New Years to get started. You will be done with this book in a few minutes. That's a good time to start.

Do not "try" or "do your best." Just get it done! If you received a billion dollars for consistent gym attendance for a month, you would make it happen. If you got to go out on a date with a Victoria Secret model for being on a diet for a month, it would suddenly become a much easier task. My point here is that if you considered it important enough, you would do it.

The programs presented here require 3-4 weekly sessions about hour long each. Yet out of 168 hours in a week, these are the 3-4 hour people desperately need in their lives. Everything seems to fall during the scheduled gym time. We are able to find 40 hours a week for work. We manage to squeeze in 10-15 years of school in our lives. But when it comes to gym, due to some mysterious reason things are just not working out.

What you see a lot is that people set hidden traps for themselves. They plan so much activities around their workouts that they end up being "forced" to skip a session. And they don't even realize they are doing it. A good telltale sign that this is what's happening is when you hear "I have too much on my plate." People would rather get a second job so they can buy fancy clothes to "appear" good than to go to the gym and ACTUALLY look good. Are we missing the point?

If you ever rode a bike, you know that the first few yards are always the hardest - it takes some effort to gain momentum. But once you have reached the desired speed, maintaining it is pretty easy. The same thing happens with working out. The first few sessions will feel like an uphill battle. You have to adjust your daily routine to schedule REGULAR training sessions. You have to find a gym and what to wear. You have to learn all the exercises while feeling like everyone around is watching (or even laughing at you). The whole time your overprotective mind is going to keep producing "legitimate" reasons for why should quit: they should accept you the way you are, you don't have to prove anything to anyone, you are going to get injured, ... It might seem overwhelming at first, but once you get pass the initial frustration, continuing to exercise will be pretty easy. The fact that you made it this far through the book is already a good sign.

Don't expect your friends and family to support you. They already convinced themselves that it simply cannot be done and will subconsciously test your commitment in the beginning. Your girlfriend will always get "in the mood" when you about to leave to the gym. Your friends will ask to skip "just this one time" and go out for a beer instead. Say "no." It might be a bit uncomfortable at first, but once you gain some momentum, they will actually respect you for staying the course.

Discipline is not always about going hardcore. Sometimes it is about being methodical. It's about sticking to the plan. It's about not attempting the weight ahead of time. It's about backing off when light training is scheduled. Some people find such self-restraint equally as hard.

Consider developing patience, consistency and persistence to be as important outcomes of training as getting bigger and stronger. Familiarize yourself with a training program and follow it to the T. If you know your mother's birthday party will be in the evening, go in the morning. If some unexpected urgent matter came up with your kid, make up on the weekend. Unless you are injured or sick, do not allow yourself to skip even one time. From what I've seen, once a single slip occurs, complete deterioration of the gym attendance follows soon after.

Allow the training to build your character. *Successful development of good work habits at the gym will carry over to other areas of your life.* Setting training goals and achieving them will give you the confidence to pursue your dreams outside of the gym.

Addendum

(Advanced Bench Press Program)

Week 1

SATURDAY – A	SUNDAY – B	TUESDAY – C	THURSDAY – D
Barbell bench press 5x6 (70%)	Back squat 5x6 (70%)	Standing barbell press 5x6 (70%)	Deadlift 5x6 (70%)
Seated dumbbell press 3x12-10	Barbell bent-over row 3x12-10	Incline dumbbell press 3x12-10	Dumbbell shrug 3x12-10
Lying EZ-bar triceps extension 3x12-10	Barbell biceps curl 3x12-10	Close grip barbell bench press 3x12-10	Leg press 3x12-10
Dip 3x12-10	Standing calf raise 3x12-10	Incline sit-up 3x12-10	Pull-up / pulldown 3x12-10

Week 2

SATURDAY – A	SUNDAY – B	TUESDAY – C	THURSDAY – D
Barbell bench press 5x5 (74%)	Back squat 5x5 (74%)	Standing barbell press 5x5 (74%)	Deadlift 5x5 (74%)
Seated dumbbell press 3x10-8	Barbell bent-over row 3x10-8	Incline dumbbell press 3x10-8	Dumbbell shrug 3x10-8
Lying EZ-bar triceps extension 3x10-8	Barbell biceps curl 3x10-8	Close grip barbell bench press 3x10-8	Leg press 3x10-8
Dip 3x10-8	Standing calf raise 3x10-8	Incline sit-up 2x12-10	Pull-up / pulldown 3x10-8

Week 3

SATURDAY – A	SUNDAY – B	TUESDAY – C	THURSDAY – D
Barbell bench press 5x4 (79%)	Back squat 5x4 (79%)	Standing barbell press 5x4 (79%)	Deadlift 5x4 (79%)
Seated dumbbell press 3x8-6	Barbell bent-over row 3x8-6	Incline dumbbell press 3x8-6	Dumbbell shrug 3x8-6
Lying triceps extension 3x8-6	Barbell biceps curl 3x8-6	Close grip barbell bench press 3x8-6	Leg press 3x8-6
Dip 3x8-6	Standing calf raise 3x8-6	Incline sit-up 1x12-10	Pull-up / pulldown 3x8-6

Week 4

SUNDAY - A	TUESDAY - B	THURSDAY - A
Barbell bench press 4x3 (85%)	Deadlift 4x5 (69%)	Barbell bench press 4x6 (65%)
Back squat 4x3 (85%)	Standing barbell military press 4x5 (69%)	Back squat 4x6 (65%)
Dip 2x8-6	Barbell bent-over row 2x8-6	Dip 2x8-6

Week 5

SUNDAY - B	TUESDAY - A	THURSDAY - B
Deadlift 4x3 (85%)	Barbell bench press 4x4 (75%)	Deadlift 4x6 (65%)
Standing barbell military press 4x3 (85%)	Back squat 4x4 (75%)	Standing barbell military press 4x6 (65%)
Barbell bent-over row 1x8-6	Dip 1x8-6	Barbell bent-over row 1x8-6

Week 6

SUNDAY - A	TUESDAY - B	THURSDAY - A
Barbell bench press 3x2 (92%)	Standing barbell military press 3x4 (75%)	Barbell bench press 3x5 (72%)
Back squat 3x2 (92%)	Deadlift 3x4 (75%)	Back squat 3x5 (72%)

Week 7

SUNDAY - B	TUESDAY - A	THURSDAY - B
Standing barbell military press 3x2 (92%)	Barbell bench press 2x3 (82%)	Standing barbell military press 1x5 (72%)
Deadlift 3x2 (92%)	Back squat 2x3 (82%)	Pull-up / pulldown 1x5

Week 8

SUNDAY	WEDNESDAY	
Barbell bench press 1RM (100%+)	Deload workout	REPEAT

- If the weight feels easy for the assigned number of reps, focus on lifting it (*concentric action*) as fast as possible, while lowering it (*eccentric action*) with approximately the same speed as you do on 1RM attempts.

Made in the USA
Monee, IL
01 December 2019